Living SMART

*Five Essential Skills to Change
Your Health Habits Forever*

Joshua C. Klapow, Ph.D.
Associate Professor
Department of Health Care Organization and Policy
South Central Center for Public Health Preparedness
University of Alabama at Birmingham
Birmingham, Alabama

and

Sheri D. Pruitt, Ph.D.
Director of Behavioral Science Integration
The Permanente Medical Group
Sacramento, California

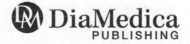

DiaMedica PUBLISHING

Visit our website at www.livingsmart.diamedicapub.com

Library of Congress Cataloging-in-Publication Data
Available from the publisher.

ISBN-13: 978-0-9793564-0-7
ISBN-10: 0-9793564-0-7

Printed in Canada

Editor: Jessica Bryan
Composition: TypeWriting

Contents

About the Authors

Joshua C. Klapow, Ph.D. is an Associate Professor in the Department of Health Care Organization and Policy at the University of Alabama at Birmingham. He received his Ph.D. in Clinical Psychology, with a specialization in Behavioral Medicine from the University of California, San Diego. Dr. Klapow has served as a behavioral science consultant to the World Health Organization, and he is the author of more than 100 professional articles, abstracts, and book chapters in the area of behavioral medicine and health psychology. He is a member of the South Central Center for Public Health Preparedness, where he serves as a mental health specialist and writes and produces "The Preparedness Minute" video series.

In addition to his academic pursuits, Dr. Klapow hosts the weekly television segments "Healthy Habits" and "The Healthy Action Minute" on the ABC affiliate in Birmingham, Alabama. He has been interviewed by a variety of national print and Internet-based media outlets including: *Tribune Media Services, Associated Press, United Press International, Reuters Health, ABC News.com, Weightwatchers.com, iVillage.com, Kiplinger's, Self, Men's Health, Women's Day, Prevention, Redbook, Shape,* and *Fitness.*

Sheri D. Pruitt, Ph.D. is a speaker, writer, and consultant in the areas of behavioral medicine and health psychology. She received her Ph.D. in clinical psychology from the University of New Mexico, and she is currently Director of Behavioral Science Integration for The Permanente Medical Group in Sacramento, California, where she uses innovative technologies and behavioral science to solve problems in the delivery of health care. Dr. Pruitt has worked as a behavioral scientist for the World Health Organization and is the principal author of two books on global strategies for the management of chronic health problems. She is the developer of an innovative, Internet-based health coaching program that provides motivation and behavioral skills training using new media technology.

Dr. Pruitt is a popular lecturer and keynote speaker in the Northern California region and frequently shares behavioral science expertise with local and national newspapers, radio, and television stations. She has provided ClearChannel Radio announcements and cable television network commercials, which have aired on NBC, CBS, ABC, WB Network, Lifetime, and MTV.

Acknowledgments

Many people have supported our efforts in writing this book; our patients, students, mentors, and colleagues have all helped to shape its contents. We are also grateful to Arlene Mickley, who helped us navigate the world of publishing.

Our mentors, Mark Slater, Ph.D., Douglas Ferraro, Ph.D., and William R. Miller, Ph.D. helped us develop as scientists and as individuals. We rely daily on the foundation of knowledge they provided.

We also acknowledge and honor the work of Jeffery Fisher, Ph.D. and William Fisher, Ph.D., whose Information-Motivation-Behavioral Skills model gave us the inspiration and empirical foundation to explain behavior change in a simpler, more intuitive way.

Special thanks to our families, who tolerated endless discussions about titles and graphics, and read numerous drafts. Josh especially thanks his wife, Julie, and his children, Maxwell and Adair. As always, Sheri thanks her parents and her husband, Steve.

Finally, many thanks to our publisher, Dr. Diana M. Schneider, who saw our "diamond in the rough" and believed in what we were trying to accomplish. We are also grateful to Jessica Bryan, our editor, for helping us preserve the scientific integrity of our work, while refining the way in which it's delivered.

*To all of us who have ever struggled
with the process of change*

Preface

We want to start by setting the record straight. Somehow, despite the many advances in medicine during the past few decades, we have taken a dangerous path when it comes to our health. Obesity is common, lifestyle-related diseases, such as diabetes, are on the increase, and many of us avoid healthy behaviors, such as following a healthy diet, exercising, taking medication properly, getting adequate sleep, not smoking, and reducing the stress in our lives. We are searching and hoping for a pill, surgery, or procedure that will make us healthy—quickly and with little effort.

When it comes to such things as a headache, an upset stomach, or a bacterial infection, often there *is* a quick fix. But we absolutely *must* stop this line of thinking when it comes to health-related lifestyles. Every step we take to improve our health requires that we change our behavior. There is no magic bullet or a way to make changes that requires nothing from us. The reality is that change requires each person to put forth some amount of effort.

A great deal is known about how to make needed changes in health-related behavior—or any other change, for that matter. Theories of behavioral change such as the "Transtheoretical Model of Behavior Change," the "Health Belief Model," the "Theory of Planned Behavior," and "Social Learning Theory" have all proposed reasonable explanations as to how and why behavior change occurs.

The problem with these theories and the impression they give to the general public is that changing behavior is either:

✔ Incredibly complicated, and dependent on a series of cognitive, emotional, and behavioral interactions that may require professional counseling, or

✔ A simple matter of common sense and self-motivation

We believe there is a lot of room between these two extremes. This book will give you a set of tools that goes beyond "common sense and motivation," without attempting to deal with the complexities of psychological treatment and advanced behavioral science. Why?—Because most of the answers to making healthy lifestyle changes can be found somewhere in between. We like the common sense, the simplicity, and the scientific foundation of the Information-Motivation-Behavioral Skills model of change developed by Jeffrey Fisher, Ph.D. and his brother, William Fisher, Ph.D. We use their model as the basis for a simple set of guiding principles that will give you the ability to change *any* health behavior or health habit.

What a powerful concept. Think about it—any health habit you want to change. This book will help you take control of your health and your life. The information it contains works with any diet, exercise, sleep, or stop-smoking program. In fact, this book will help you change any behavior that has a negative impact on your well-being, health-related or not.

The essential tools you need to make change happen are the SMART skills, which underlie all successful behavior change. SMART is an acronym that can help you remember these key behavior change skills:

S et a goal
M onitor your progress
A rrange your world for success
R ecruit a support team
T reat yourself

Living SMART is based on the idea that your health and wellbeing is determined mostly by what you do or don't do *every day*. Regardless of the severity of your situation, the history of the problems or how complicated the the issue may feel, your success is determined by the actions you take. This set of principles will guide you through the process of change. Living SMART means:

✔ Having the skill to change what you need to change and what you want to change
✔ Not being perfect, but doing the "right" behaviors more days than not
✔ Having the confidence that you can succeed

If you keep the acronym SMART in mind and use the skills it represents, you will be well on your way to making lasting changes in your behavior.

In our work, we talk to patients, health care professionals, executive boards, human resource professionals, local reading clubs, college students, and many others. Two things have become clear to us from these experiences. First, people are pleasantly surprised to find that changing their behavior doesn't have to be an arduous task. Second, they are usually quite busy and welcome help and guidance with the change process. We took these two facts to heart in writing this book.

Living SMART can be read in sections. You don't need to read it from cover to cover to get what you need. Read Part I: "What It Takes to Change Your Health" if you want to understand the basic principles that underlie making any change in behavior. "When Life Gets Tough" in Part III (Chapter 11) can help you when you are having problems sticking with the changes you've made, as everyone does. If you need a quick tip, something to keep your motivation levels up, take a look at the "Action Tips" found in each chapter, or review them on our Web site: www.livingsmart.diamedicapub.com.

Sometimes we need a little extra guidance to "jump start" our progress towards change. Having a game plan or strategy is critical. Diet, exercise, taking medications properly, and getting adequate sleep are common health-related behaviors that have a huge impact on overall health and well being. Because these are such common issues, we'll give you a strategy for making changes in each of them. The information in Part II "Your Game Plans" will help you start making changes in any or all of these areas.

We are excited about this book, and enthusiastic about helping you become as healthy as possible. But remember, it's what you do or don't do every day that affects your health more than anything else. Take control now and become healthier starting today. Here's to your health!

Joshua C. Klapow, Ph.D.
Sheri D. Pruitt, Ph.D.

Introduction

Stop Wishing and Start Living SMART

Congratulations on wanting to be healthy. You are taking an important step by reading this book, which will tell you exactly how to change your behavior to improve your health.

The Problem: Our Health

You've probably noticed we're in big trouble in our country. Obesity is at an all-time high, diabetes is skyrocketing, and only half of us take our medications the way our doctors prescribe. People are still smoking, drinking too much, and sleeping too little. We're more stressed out and more sedentary than ever before. How can this be? We have the most sophisticated healthcare system in the world—the best doctors, the most medications. Why are Americans so unhealthy?

The Reason: Our Behavior

We are the reason that we're unhealthy. Every one of us has some level of control over our own health, but we've been ignoring the root of so many of our health problems: our behavior.

With all the talk about increasing health care costs, chronic disease, and diseases caused by lifestyle, there has been little discussion about how people can change their habits to improve their health. We've heard that health habits are important and that we *should* change them, but *how*?

The degree to which our behavior affects our health often surprises people. In our work as psychologists, people often ask us about genetics. They say: "Don't genes determine a person's health?" Genetics *are* important. Your genes set the stage for how behavior affects your health. Think of your genes as the hand of cards you have been dealt. If you have a good set of genes, you can do unhealthy things and still live well. If you were born with a set of genes that make you susceptible to health issues, you need to make the effort to be as healthy as possible, because the cards are stacked against you.

Consider heart disease. It has a genetic component, but behavior can dramatically influence its development. If you have genes that make you susceptible to heart disease and you smoke, drink too much, and never exercise, what will happen? You'll most likely develop serious heart problems. If you have the same genes and you keep your weight in check, exercise, drink in moderation, and don't smoke, you may never have heart problems. We can say the same thing about diabetes, obesity, and many other conditions.

Changing Behavior: It's Not Just about Being Motivated

You've been told to get motivated and make changes in your lifestyle, right? Not so fast! As psychologists, we see patients every day who are frustrated and sick, and getting sicker. They've been told to change their diet, relax, exercise, and stop smoking and drinking. When they fail to make these necessary changes, they're told they lack motivation. People look everywhere for answers about how to change: the Internet, self-help books, magazines, and infomercials, but they can't find the solution.

There *are* scientific answers to this problem. Psychologists and others who study human behavior have known for decades what it takes to successfully change health habits. However, the answers they've come up with haven't been readily available to the people who need them—or when the answers are available, they have been presented in ways that are difficult to understand and apply to daily life.

We All Need a Healthier Lifestyle

Whether you want to start an exercise program, begin to diet, quit smoking, reduce stress, get more organized, spend less money, or make any other lifestyle change, many books and programs are available. The sheer number of different strategies can be overwhelming, but there is a common thread. All of the diet and exercise books, the stop-smoking programs, and the organizational and financial strategies require that you change your behavior in order to succeed. Unfortunately, these tools often lack instructions on *how* to change your behavior. Most of the information about improving lifestyle focuses only on *what* to change, rarely on *how* to change. This is the missing piece that makes the difference between success and failure when it comes to changing health-related behavior. The information in *Living SMART* works with any diet, exercise, or stop-smoking program. It gives you what the others do not: a simple approach to change any behavior that has a negative impact on your health and lifestyle

Myth and Reality

Many false claims, myths, and erroneous assumptions have helped to create a way of thinking that is counterproductive; for example:

✔ **Myth:** If I just want to badly enough, I can make improvements in my health.

✔ **Truth:** This is the reason people fail. Motivation can only take you so far; it goes up and it goes down. You can't rely on it alone. Without the skills to make the changes you desire, you will not succeed in the long run.

✔ **Myth:** This behavior change stuff doesn't apply to me. My problem is more complicated.

✔ **Truth:** Anyone who wants to be healthier needs to change their habits. Regardless of the severity of your problems or your level of physical impairment, improving your health requires doing some things and not doing others. Whether it's taking medication, following your doctor's recommendations, or monitoring blood pressure, you will have to do something differently than you have done before.

✔ **Myth:** Changing behavior is just common sense.

✔ **Truth:** Our approach is so straightforward and so simple that people think it's not powerful. In reality, you can change any behavior if you have the right information and some motivation, and use the SMART skills. If you are struggling, you are probably missing one or more of the basic principles of change outlined in this book.

✔ **Myth:** I tried this before and it didn't work.

✔ **Truth:** You either didn't use the principles and skills, or—as is more often the case—you used them for a period of time, hit a roadblock, and then stopped. Living healthier does not mean being perfect. It means adopting healthy habits more days than not. If everyone were to have this perspective, we would all enjoy better health.

✔ **Myth:** I really want to be healthy; I just don't have the motivation.

✔ **Truth:** If you *want* to be healthy, then you already have some level of motivation. You may not have enough to carry you through to reach your goal right now, but you are definitely motivated enough to get started.

✔ **Myth:** If I just understood what caused my bad habits, I could change them.

✔ **Truth:** Understanding how your habits developed, and why they developed, is important because it can keep you from repeating a destructive pattern. However, understanding why your bad habits developed is not enough to help you change them.

Living healthier means adopting a simple set of principles and skills, and using them to guide your behavior more often than not. No one is perfect.

Okay—the myths are behind us. Are you ready to live a healthier life? Let's Go!

The Icons for Important Themes

Our goal in writing this book was to make it as simple, straightforward, and useful as possible. Thus, we have included pictures as well as words to communicate efficiently and signal important themes. The icons found throughout the book are illustrated below.

 This icon signals research findings, scientific principles, or technical terms.

 This icon signals an interactive exercise that requires your response.

 This icon signals key points and our recommendations.

Action Tips You Can Use

What you do or don't do *every day* affects your health more than anything else. With all the skills and strategies we outline in this book, with all the "tricks and tips" we offer, being successful in creating a healthy lifestyle ultimately comes down to what you *do* on a daily basis. It's up to you to take positive action, because a healthy action a day *will* help you become healthier. Each day, ideally in the morning, read and follow one of the Action Tips found throughout the book.

These tips are intended to motivate you, to give you something to sink your teeth into. You'll find that you *can* make a difference in your health habits on a daily basis by using them.

PART I

What It Takes to Change Your Health

*Y*ou have to start somewhere—you need a base from which you can begin to work. This section lays out the principles you need in order to understand what goes into making changes in your behavior. The ideas presented here are drawn from the work of Jeffery Fisher, Ph.D. and William Fisher, Ph.D., whose Information-Motivation-Behavioral Skills model gave us the inspiration and empirical foundation to explain behavior change in a simpler, more intuitive way.

This section will be your foundation for *any* change you wish to make. Once you have read it you will have what you need to decide whether you are ready to make a change, determine specific barriers that may be keeping you from succeeding at change, move forward with goal-focused change, and maintain the changes you make. Of all the sections of the book, this is the most critical and the most powerful. Learn the principles in this section and you *will* succeed at making changes and living SMART.

1

Let's Get Started

At one time or another, most of us have tried to improve our health by changing our behavior, often without success. Maybe you've tried to stop smoking, lose weight, or exercise regularly. If you haven't been successful yet, don't be too hard on yourself. True behavior change requires three important components. We call them "The What," "The Want," and "The How." Chances are you're simply missing one of them. When it comes to changing behavior, most people fall into one of three groups, or "change types:"

What Is Your "Change Type?"

1. *Uninformed:* "I don't know what to do to be healthy." Do you know *what* you need to do to feel your best? For example, are you aware that exercising, eating right, and following your doctor's recommendations are good for 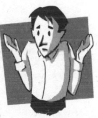 your health? Most people answer "yes" to this question. If your answer is "yes," move on to the next category. If your answer is "no," you are "uninformed," but

you can easily get the information about what you need to do to be healthy.

2. *Unmotivated:* "I don't want to do any-thing differently in order to improve my health." Do you *want* to behave in a way that will ensure that you are healthy and feel your best? Most people answer "yes" to this question—it's the "I know exer-cise is good for me and I want to do it" category. Move on to the third category if you answered "yes."

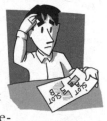

If you answered "no," you probably already know all about exercise, and understand that being active has great health benefits, but you just don't feel like exer-cising. You don't want to do anything differently to get more activity into your daily routine, although you know it would make you feel better. If so, this book is not for you—but in all likelihood you wouldn't be reading this book if you fall into this category!

3. *Unskilled:* "I don't know how to make changes in my behavior." You know *what* health behaviors are good for you, and you *want* to make those behaviors part of your life, but you just can't seem to *do* it. People in this cate-gory lack the skills they need to make effective lifestyle changes. Do you know how to make healthy behaviors part of your everyday life? If your answer is "no" or "I'm not sure," you are similar to most of us. Few peo-ple know how to incorporate healthy behaviors into their lifestyles, even though they understand that mak-

ing changes will help them feel better and they want to make them.

The typical response of health professionals is to tell clients over and over again that exercise (or another healthy behavior) is good for them, or that they simply need to be more motivated. However, neither of these responses seems to help people change.

These categories don't only apply to exercise. They work for virtually any health-related behavior. People usually fall into one of the three categories no matter what behavior they want to change, including dieting, smoking, taking medication, wearing a seat belt, or checking their blood pressure on a regular basis. In this chapter, you will learn the basic principles for making healthy lifestyle changes.

The Principles of Change

The ability to change your behavior in order to create a healthier lifestyle comes down to three critical factors: knowing what to do, wanting to do it, and knowing how to do it. It's really as simple as it sounds. You need The What, The Want, and The How to make any behavior change.

The What:

The What is information. You need to know what changes to make in order to reach your health goal; for example, what exercise, what food, or what medications and at what doses.

The Want:

The Want is motivation. You must want to change, plain and simple.

The How:

The How includes the skills you need to be able to change. You need to know how to make changes in your behavior so you can reach your goal. Many of us are missing these essential skills.

Changing Your Health:
The What, The Want, The How

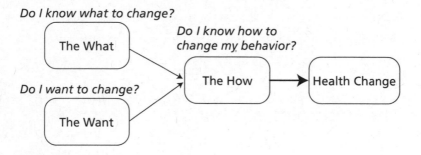

Research has shown that changing health behavior requires more than motivation—information and skills are also necessary.

In our society, we make two big assumptions about changing health behaviors. We believe that people who succeed do so because they want to, and that those who fail just aren't motivated—or we think that if we know what behaviors we need to practice (such as dieting, exercising, reducing stress, or stopping smoking), and are motivated to do them, we will be successful at making changes.

If these assumptions are true, you have to wonder whether we have a country filled with uninformed, unmotivated people. Maybe so, but we believe there is another explanation. Think about your exercise habits for a minute and then answer these questions.

1. Have you heard that exercising three to five times a week, for at least 30 minutes, is good for your health?
   YES   NO

2. Do you want exercise to be a part of your lifestyle?
   YES   NO

3. Do you exercise three to five times per week for 30 minutes or more, and have done so consistently for the past 6 months?
   YES   NO

Three Simple Steps to Change

 Any time you want to make a health change, all you need to do is determine which of the three ingredients (The What, The Want, or The How) is missing. Ask yourself these questions:

1. *The What:* Do you know exactly what to change, and how to get the information you need to make it happen: for example, what exercise do I need to do, what food should I eat, or what medications should I take and at what doses?

2. *The Want:* Do you really want to make the change?

3. *The How:* Do you know how to change your behavior to reach your goal?

Where Do I Start?

Next, use your answers to these questions to jump-start your behavioral change. If you answered "no" to question # 1, you need to gather information. Chapter 2 will be useful in helping you find it. If you answered "no" to question # 2, then you need more motivation. Chapter 3 will give you some tips on this. Finally, if you answered "no" to question # 3, you need to learn *how* to change your behavior. Chapter 4 has the answers. It really is that simple.

SMART Skills—The Key to "The How"

The core principle of this book is that you need to develop what we call "SMART" skills to make the change happen. SMART is an acronym for these five essential skills:

S	et a goal
M	onitor your progress
A	rrange your world for success
R	ecruit a support team
T	reat yourself

Throughout this book, we'll explain each step in detail. Are you ready to get started?

ACTION TIP
Exercise for People Who Hate Exercise

We all know that daily exercise is good for our health. But what if you just hate it? What if you can't stand the thought of jogging, lifting weights, or doing aerobics? Try these suggestions:

✔ Identify one small physical activity that you can do without much effort. Maybe you could walk up and down the stairs every day, or walk for 5 minutes around the neighborhood. The easier the activity, the better.

✔ Write down what you plan to do and post it on the fridge.

✔ Commit to doing this activity for one week. At the end of the week, decide if you want to continue and, hopefully, do more.

Once you engage in a small amount of activity on a regular basis, it's easy to gradually increase your efforts. With time it will develop into a daily exercise routine.

2
The What: Know Exactly What Needs to Change

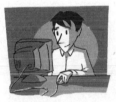Information is crucial when making any change. You need it to get started. If you don't know what you need to change, all the motivation and behavioral skills in the world won't help you. Information is without a doubt the easiest of the three ingredients to obtain. When it comes to exercise, diet, stress management, diabetes care, obesity, smoking—you name it—a wealth of information is available.

If you're reading this, you probably already know what change you need to make. However, people tend to focus all of their efforts on getting more and more information. They assume that the more information they have about making changes, the more likely they are to make them. This is simply not so.

Time and again, research has shown that information alone is not a powerful enough tool to change health behaviors. Smokers know that smoking is bad for their health, but they continue to smoke anyway. People who are overweight know they should shed the extra pounds, but they remain heavy. We are bombarded with information about health—we all know what to do. If information were enough, we would all be totally healthy.

Any information you gather must be reliable and useful. The *quality* of the information is important, not the *quantity*. A quick and easy way to organize your sources is to break them down into categories, as we've done here.

Sources of Information

People

Ask your doctor about any issues related to your health. Whether the topic is exercise, diet, blood-sugar monitoring, preventive tests, or psychological problems and counseling, your doctor's job is to support you in your quest for better health. Realize, however, that in today's healthcare setting your doctor may not have the time to provide you with a comprehensive education on all health topics. Rather, she may refer you to another healthcare professional or to another source of information. Either way, consulting with your doctor about lifestyle changes is a good way to begin.

Prepare yourself before you go to the doctor. Remember, you may only have 10 minutes, or less. Prepare for the visit by doing the following:

✔ Write your questions on a piece of paper and take it with you to the office visit.

✔ Organize the questions in order of importance. You may not have time to ask them all, so this will ensure that the most important ones are answered.

✔ When you call for an appointment, tell the doctor or office staff that you have some specific questions about lifestyle changes.

✔ Bring a pen and paper to take notes.

Written Information

The number of books, magazines, reports, and Internet sources on health is overwhelming. No one source is the most accurate, up-to-date, or reliable. When it comes to analyzing written resources, follow these general rules:

✔ *Credibility.* The information should come from a respected institution or organization. Here are just a few examples:

- Universities, such as Johns Hopkins, Harvard, or UCLA
- Government agencies, such as the National Institutes of Health/National Library of Medicine, Centers for Disease Control, and the Department of Health and Human Services
- Disease-specific organizations, such as the American Heart Association or American Cancer Society
- Healthcare systems, such as The Mayo Clinic or Kaiser Permanente

✔ *Timeliness.* Look at the date of publication to make sure that the information is current. In general, it's best to collect information that is no more than 5 years old.

✔ *Consistency.* Check to see that the information is consistent in a variety of sources. Conflicting views may pop up, but the information should be similar.

✔ *Trustworthiness.* If it sounds too good to be true, it probably is. Use common sense when evaluating information. Just because a publication uses terms you don't understand, it doesn't mean you can't grasp the overall message. Words such as "miracle," "instant," and "guaranteed" should be warning flags.

Mass Media

The same rules apply to television and radio. The source should be credible, the information should be consistent, and the claims should be reasonable. It's important to note that television and radio sources of health information can be incredibly brief. A 30-second public service announcement, a 3-minute news report, or a 10-minute radio segment may not give the whole story. While the information may be accurate, it probably won't give you the whole picture. Think of radio and television as good starting points from which to gather facts or ideas for further pursuit.

The following table will help you in your quest for information. There are many other resources available about all types of health topics, but these will help jump-start your research process.

Resources

Nutrition	U.S. Department of Agriculture: www.health.gov/dietarybooklines *Guidelines* and *Using the Dietary Guidelines* are available from the Consumer Information Center. Order online or call (888) 878-3256.
Exercise	The President's Council on Physical Fitness and Sports: www.fitness.gov For more information, call (202) 690-9000.
Smoking	American Lung Association: www.lungusa.org/ To speak to a lung health professional, contact the American Lung Association Call Center at (800) 548-8252.
Substance Abuse	National Institute on Drug Abuse: www.drugabuse.gov/ For more information, contact the National Clearinghouse for Alcohol and Drug Information at (800) 729-6686.
Cancer Prevention	Centers for Disease Control: www.cdc.gov/cancer For more information, call the Centers for Disease Control at (888) 842-6355.

HIV/STD Prevention	National Prevention Information Network: www.cdcnpin.org For more information, call (800) 458-5231.
Diabetes	National Diabetes Education Program: www.ndep.nih.gov/ Call (800) 438-5383 to order education materials for consumers and healthcare providers.
Heart Disease	American Heart Association: www.americanheart.org For more information, contact the American Heart Association at (800) AHA-USA-1 or (800) 242-8721.
Obesity	U.S. Department of Health and Human Services: www.smallstep.gov For more information, call (877) 696-6775.
Sleep	National Sleep Foundation: www.sleepfoundation.org For more information, call (202) 347-3471.
Medication	American Society of Health System Pharmacists: www.medicationsafety.com For more information call (301) 657-3000.

Getting the information you need should be simple. Now, let's move on to the more challenging components of change: The Want and The How.

ACTION TIP
Stack the Odds in Your Favor

Having a healthy lifestyle can reduce the risk of everything from cancer to heart disease, but sticking with it is often easier said than done. When you're trying to create a new health habit, it often feels as if the odds are stacked against you. The trick is to change your environment so things are more in your favor. You can do this by making small changes in the world around you.

If you want to exercise in the morning, have your gym clothes ready to go and your alarm clock set. If you want to make sure you don't cheat on your diet, get rid of the cookies. To increase your chances of not smoking, throw out the ashtrays and lighters, not just the cigarettes. So, take charge of the odds. Look around and see how you could modify your environment to ensure success.

3

The Want: Decide Whether You Want to Change

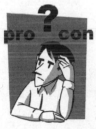 Motivation—or lack thereof—is the great stumbling block. "If only I were motivated enough, I could do this." Negative thoughts, self-defeating beliefs, and a history of failed attempts at making changes, all contribute to decreased self-esteem, efficiency, and motivation. Why do you have negative thoughts and beliefs? What is driving them? Although the answers to these questions are important, not having answers doesn't mean you can't change your unwanted behaviors. Many books focus on the origin of self-defeating thoughts, attitudes, and beliefs; countless magazine articles focus on why you think the way you do. These sources can help, but they may not be completely necessary. We often spend so much time focusing on why we are the way we are that we don't focus on moving forward. Motivation is complicated, but we can simplify it by getting right to the heart of the question. Ask yourself, "Do I want to make a change in my behavior?" In other words, do you *want* to do something differently to improve your health?

If your answer to this question is: "No, I don't want to make a change to improve my health," you're not going to make the change successfully. That's it. Sometimes people are not ready emotionally or psychologically to do things differently. If you are not ready to change, nothing can force you to do it. However, if you are even slightly motivated, you *can* be a success. With just a small amount of motivation, you can take action that may boost your level of motivation even further and maintain it during the change process.

Evaluate your level of motivation using this scale:

1	2	3	4	5	6	7	8	9	10
A little									Strongly
motivated									motivated

Your motivation level may be higher or lower depending on the activity, the time, and the setting. The most important thing is to have *some* motivation. Once you have it, you can give it a boost when necessary. This chapter includes several strategies to help you do just that. So, stop worrying about motivation—you'll have enough to succeed.

Think about Your Future

What if you aren't sure you are motivated enough to make a change? What if you think it's not worth it to be healthier? Stop for a minute and think about your future. If you don't change your health habits, will you still be here 5 years from now? Will you be in any kind of shape to work, go on vacation, and enjoy life? How will you feel? What will you look like? Your future and your ability to do the things you enjoy in that future is determined in large part by what you do today, tomorrow, the next day, and so on. Do you want to be healthy 5 years from now? If you're not sure, ask yourself these questions and write down the answers:

✔ What behavior are you most likely to change to improve your health? _____.

✔ What made you select this particular behavior? _____.

✔ How would you feel if you were to make this change? _____.

✔ What else would be different about you? _____ _____.

✔ What behavior have you been able to change in the past? _____.
Next, imagine yourself 5 years from now:

✔ If my behavior stays the same, I will feel _____ _____.

✔ If I keep doing exactly what I am doing now, I will look
_____.

✔ If I don't change a thing, my health will be _____
_____.

Imagine your loved ones 5 years from now:

✔ If my behavior stays the same, it will affect my loved
ones by _____.

✔ If my behavior stays the same, my loved ones may react
by _____.

By taking the time to answer these questions, most people will be reminded of why they set out to make changes in the first place. Simple as it seems, this little reminder can really boost your level of motivation. So, if you ever find your motivation slipping, repeat this exercise.

The Pros and Cons of Change

There are advantages and disadvantages to changing any behavior, and it's important to consider both when you're trying to get motivated. For example, think about eating ice cream every night as a midnight snack. This is a behavior that some people want to change because they want to lose weight. Consider the pros and cons of continuing or stopping this behavior:

Behavior: Eating ice cream every night

Continuing the Behavior:	
Pros	**Cons**
If I continue eating ice cream, I will continue to enjoy the cool, creamy, sweet taste that I love so much.	If I continue eating ice cream every night, I'll keep gaining weight.
Changing the Behavior:	
Pros	**Cons**
If I cut down on ice cream, I'll feel more in control of my eating habits.	If I reduce my ice cream intake, I'll feel deprived.

Name the behavior you want to change:

_____

_____.

Next, apply the same "pros and cons" strategy to determine the advantages and disadvantages of making this particular behavioral change.

Behavior I Want to Change: _____

Continuing the Behavior:	
Pros	Cons

Changing the Behavior:	
Pros	Cons

How Important Is Change? Can I Do It?

Finally, using the scales below, rate how important it is for you to make the behavioral change you're considering and how confident you are that you will succeed:

1. How important is it that I make the change?

1	2	3	4	5	6	7	8	9	10

Not
important

Extremely
important

2. What would make this behavioral change more important?

_____

_____

3. Am I confident I can make the change?

1	2	3	4	5	6	7	8	9	10

Not confident
at all

Extremely
confident

4. What would make you more confident?
   (Circle yes or no.)

More information?	Yes	No
Smaller changes?	Yes	No
Help making the change?	Yes	No
More reasons to change?	Yes	No

After answering these questions, you have probably discovered a number of reasons for changing or refusing to change an unhealthy behavior. You've probably realized that your emotions play a significant role in your decision to make the change. Thinking about changing a behavior can bring up a variety of feelings, including anger, fear of failure, and anxiety. While change can be difficult and stressful, consider the consequences of refusing to change. What are you doing today to become the healthy person you envision yourself being in the future? How long can you afford to wait before making the change?

A Shortcut around Motivation

Do you have thoughts similar to these?

✔ "I just don't have any willpower."
✔ "If I only knew why I undermine myself."
✔ "All of my problems stem from my mother."

This kind of "self-talk" is a psychological merry-go-round that can keep you from changing your behavior. However, there may be a way to get off this ride. It's possible to change your emotions and your level of motivation by first changing your behavior, because changing behavior has a way of changing thinking.

It's difficult to think of yourself as failing at exercise when you are walking for 30 minutes, four times a week. It's hard to say you're not confident in your ability to diet when you have cut down on the amount of sweets you eat.

ACTION TIP
Unclutter Your Life

Ugh—clutter—it's everywhere and it seems to grow and grow. Most of us want to get organized, but it can be stressful and overwhelming. Where do you start? How long will it take? The key to getting clutter out of your life is to start small, very small.

For clutter at home, don't try to organize your whole house or even a whole room. Instead, pick one small section of a room to organize. Then pick a day and a set amount of time to get the job done. When you've got the first section done, pick another. Same thing at work; tackle office clutter one corner at a time.

Remember, it took weeks or maybe even years to accumulate that clutter. Tackling the job one section at time will make the task much more manageable and a lot less stressful.

When you participate in the behaviors you want to adopt, you will no longer believe you are a failure.

Beating Negative Thoughts

You can be sailing along and, all of a sudden, it happens. Some small setback occurs in your diet, exercise program, or management of your blood pressure, and then the flood of negative thoughts comes. Negative thoughts will dampen your motivation, but they don't have to mean the end of your success. You can stop them before they take over. Here is a simple three-step strategy to manage negative thoughts:

1. *Notice when you have negative thoughts.* Negative thoughts usually follow a slip-up in maintaining a changed behavior—you cheated on your diet or you missed your workout. Take a minute to write down what's going through your mind. What are your thoughts? Maybe you're thinking negatively: "I have no self-control" or "I'm not disciplined enough to do this."

2. *Turn the thought into an action.* Once you've caught the negative thought and written it down, repeat it out loud, but imagine that someone else is saying it to you. For example, imagine that someone said, "You have no self-control" or "You're just not disciplined enough." As silly as this may sound, you will be more likely to stick up for yourself by picturing someone else saying the words.

3. *Defend yourself.* Is it really true that you have no self-control? Chances are this negative thought isn't 100% accurate. Write down as many situations as you can think of that prove this negative thought is wrong. Think about the times when you have shown self-control. Also, think about other explanations for why you slipped up this time. The bottom line is to defend yourself against the negative thought.

This exercise won't keep you from having negative thoughts, and it won't prevent occasional slip-ups, but it can help keep negative thoughts from taking over and ruining your efforts. By catching negative thoughts as they come up, and defeating them, you will be more likely to stay motivated and stay on track

Still Not Motivated?

After going through these exercises, most people are reminded of why they want to make changes. They have the motivation to do something differently. If you've read this section and gone through the exercises, and you still have no motivation—then we are concerned. Changing does require time and effort, so it's possible you truly lack the motivation to be healthier. Perhaps you feel you'll be okay without making changes. Perhaps you simply don't want to change your life or your health. You make the choice. The timing may not be right.

However, most people are ready to take the next step: learning the SMART skills you will need to make changes in your health behavior. The next chapter will help you do just that.

ACTION TIP
Optimism

Did you know that being optimistic can improve your health? Research has shown that optimistic people tend to have stronger immune systems, are less prone to cancer, and tend to live longer following a heart attack. The good news is that optimism is a behavior that can be learned. Try this exercise:

Every night at bedtime, write down three things that went really well during the day. They can be small things such as: "My kids were cooperative and gave me a hug," or big things: "Today I got a raise" or "I got promoted."

Next to each event, write down the reasons *why* the good thing happened. For example, maybe your children were cooperative because they went to bed earlier the night before. Doing this exercise will help you spend part of your day thinking about and focusing on positive events in your life, and you will end your day on an optimistic note. Over time, you will begin to increase your level of optimism.

Why not start being more optimistic—it's good for you, and it will benefit the people around you, too.

4

The How: SMART Skills to Change Your Behavior

Remember the five SMART skills:

S	et a goal
M	onitor your progress
A	rrange your world for success
R	ecruit a support team
T	reat yourself

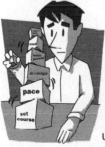 Here comes the part that gets overlooked, swept under the carpet, or written off as "just common sense." The secret is that for most people these skills are the key to being successful. When they fail to use the skills, they struggle; when they use them, they succeed. There's nothing magic about this—it's based on the results from decades of behavioral science research. The problem is that people don't use the skills because they *are* so practical and straightforward. Please hear us loud and clear on this one—if you know what needs to change *and* you are moti-

vated to make the change, with these five skills *you will* succeed.

Why the acronym SMART? This acronym is of great importance because, without even trying, you will be able to remember the set of skills that are needed to make any change. If you learn and adopt these skills, you will be able to change any behavior. As we have seen, even those who are highly motivated to change often fail because changing is more than simply wanting to change; it also requires information and a set of essential skills.

Behavioral skills are nothing more than techniques that increase your chances of changing your behavior. Think about learning them in the same way as you might think about learning how to play a sport or enjoy a hobby. For example, to play basketball you need to be able to run, jump, dribble, shoot, and pass. You may know quite a bit about the sport of basketball, but without these basic skills you won't be successful in playing it. In addition, you can't be successful at basketball if you only know how to dribble or pass. To play the sport you need *all* of the skills.

Apply this concept to making lifestyle changes. If you want to eat differently, exercise, stop smoking, reduce stress, or make any other change, you need a *set* of skills to be successful. This is where the SMART skills come in. These techniques must be used together to achieve change. They will help you make any change you want, but only if you apply all of them. It's that simple. The first SMART skill is:

S et a Goal

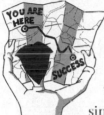

Think for a moment about a trip or vacation you took recently. Did you decide where you wanted to go before you left? Did you decide how you were going to get there? Of course you did! Making plans is simple common sense. Basic plans such as these are also the foundation of goal-setting. Goal-setting involves establishing where you want to go and how you plan to get there. As the saying goes, "Most people don't plan to fail, they fail to plan."

How do you set the *right* goal? Goals such as "I want to exercise daily," "I want to go on a diet," or "I want to get more sleep," are good ideas, but they are not specific enough. When you think about setting goals, keep two words in mind: "observable" and "measurable." Take a second and think about this. It's difficult to observe "exercise," but you can easily observe specific types of exercise such as walking, running, swimming, or weight lifting. You can't observe diet, but you can observe the specific foods you consume. You can't observe getting more sleep, but you can observe the number of hours of sleep you get each night. By making your goals observable, they automatically become measurable. The basic idea is that if you can see it, you can measure it. Once your goals are measurable you can chart them, keep track of them, and—bingo!—you have a road map from your starting point to your end point.

ACTION TIP
Stay on Top of Your Healthy Assets

What do balancing your checkbook and staying healthy have in common? We all know that balancing our checkbook helps us keep track of money so we don't overspend. The same principle applies to virtually any health habit. By tracking your health habits, you'll automatically increase your chances for a healthier life.

Writing down what you do will dramatically increase your chances of sticking with a diet or exercise program, or remembering to take your medication. Every time you exercise, write down what you did, the day you did it, and the amount of time you exercised. If you are dieting, simply jot down everything you eat in a notebook you keep with you. If you are taking medications, keep a calendar to track the times you take it. The same applies to any health habit you are trying to change.

 We call the observable and measurable behaviors you want to accomplish "target behaviors."

One of the biggest problems people have in trying to change their behavior is that they don't specify their target behaviors. Think about brushing your teeth. Seems simple enough, right? Now think about teaching a 3-year-old child how to brush his teeth. Remember, this is as foreign to him as learning a new language might be to you. How would you do it? You could just "show" him by modeling it. But that usually doesn't work. A better approach would be to break down the simple task of brushing his teeth into even smaller steps; for example:

1. Unscrew the top of the toothpaste.
2. Pick up the toothbrush.
3. Hold the toothbrush in one hand and squeeze the toothpaste onto the toothbrush with the other hand.
4. Put the toothpaste down.
5. Turn on the water.
6. Put the toothbrush under the water for 3 seconds.
7. Raise the toothbrush to your mouth.
8. Brush each tooth in a slow, circular motion.
9. Spit out the excess toothpaste into the sink.
10. Rinse off the toothbrush.
11. Fill a small cup with water.
12. Take a small amount of water into your mouth and swish it around.
13. Spit out the water.
14. Turn the water off.
15. Wipe your mouth.
16. Replace the top of the toothpaste tube cap.
17. Put the toothpaste and toothbrush away.

The simpler the behavior, the greater the chance you have of accomplishing it. Brushing the teeth maybe confusing for a 3-year-old, but each one of these 17 tasks alone is quite manageable. Break the act down into simple tasks, and the child will succeed.

Let's now bring this concept back to lifestyle changes. Adults, too, need help with breaking big tasks into manageable pieces. Below are some examples of general goals and corresponding target behaviors that are observable and measurable:

General Goal	Target Behavior
1. I want to eat better.	I will eat five servings of fruits or vegetables each day.
2. I want to exercise more.	I will walk every day, starting at 15 minutes a day and increasing by 5 minutes a week until I am walking 30 minutes each day.
3. I need to relax.	I will practice relaxation exercises for 10 minutes, three times a day (before breakfast, after lunch, and before bedtime).

To make any lifestyle change, you must start with a goal. Chances are that goal will be too broad, at first. So, break your goal down into its smallest target behaviors.

Let's practice the first step toward reaching your goals. Below, write down three of your general health goals and then break each one down into target behaviors that you can see and measure.

General Health Goal	Target Behaviors
1. _____	_____
_____	_____
_____	_____
2. _____	_____
_____	_____
_____	_____
3. _____	_____
_____	_____
_____	_____

 Your goals should be observable, measurable, and not too far-reaching.

So how do you decide the *level* at which your goals should be? Most people have a tendency to shoot for the stars, even when they break their goals down into target behaviors. If you want to be able to exercise 5 days a week, you already know that you must break the exercise down into specific target behaviors. Let's say your target behavior is to lift weights for 20 minutes and walk for 20 minutes, 5 days a week. Should you start out at this level? Think about what might happen if you do.

You make it through the full workout on the first day. You're pretty tired and wake up the next day feeling sore, fatigued, and generally worn out. What are you likely to do? You probably feel too tired to go back and do it again. You decide to skip a day, because you still have 5 days left in the week to get in four more work-outs. You work out again the next day, but you're still sore and unable to complete the 20-minute walking por-tion of the workout. The next morning, you wake up fatigued and still sore.

Where are you at this point? You've successfully com-pleted one workout, skipped another, and partially com-pleted a second. *You are not on a good path.* Your workouts are already becoming spotty, and each one is followed by unpleasant consequences (feeling sore and fatigued).

Behaviors that do not produce consistently positive results are not likely to be repeated. To make your new behavior a habit, you need to guarantee that each workout has a good chance of being a success. This is where *pacing* comes in. Pacing is simply the act of gradually increasing the intensity, duration, and frequency of a desired behav-ior in a way that maximizes your chances of success.

Whether your goal is a 40-minute workout or the elimi-nation of excess salt from your diet, pacing can help you accomplish it. The rule of thumb is that making gradual changes toward your goal are more likely to lead to success than one giant change. For any given health behavior, ask

ACTION TIP
Pace Yourself

Developing *any* health habit starts with setting a specific goal. But, even if your goal is specific, you can get into trouble if it isn't reachable right from the start. An hour of running every day, or trying to lose 30 pounds in 2 weeks, may be more than you can handle. If you can't do the behavior consistently, you'll never reach the goal. The trick is to pace yourself.

Using exercise as an example, let's say you're absolutely sure you can accomplish 30 minutes of walking. Take that amount and cut it in half for the first week. For the first week, you will walk for no more and no less than 15 minutes. For each subsequent week, add 5 more minutes to the workout, no more and no less.

At the end of 4 weeks, you will have reached your goal, and you also will have been exercising for 4 weeks. Research shows that, in order to exercise regularly, you must develop the exercise habit *before* you develop the physical conditioning. You accomplish two things with this pacing schedule: You are practicing the behavior consistently and you are giving yourself the best chance at success each time you practice it. Those two accomplishments are absolutely critical for developing healthy habits.

yourself this question: "What portion of the behavior am I absolutely sure I can do successfully?" or "What target behavior am I sure I can achieve?"

 Remember, it's better to start small and be successful over the long term than to shoot for the stars and miss.

M onitor Your Progress

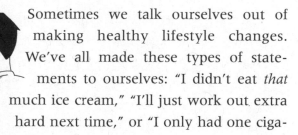 Sometimes we talk ourselves out of making healthy lifestyle changes. We've all made these types of statements to ourselves: "I didn't eat *that* much ice cream," "I'll just work out extra hard next time," or "I only had one cigarette yesterday."

Our minds are powerful and great at helping us rationalize unhealthy choices. Changing your lifestyle can be challenging enough, and excuses seem to slip in if the changes are not countable, observable, and tracked. Does this mean you aren't motivated? Does it mean that you're a failure? No, it just means that you are trying to break one habit and start another, and your mind is trying to keep things the same as they have always been.

 "Self-monitoring" is a technical term for keeping a written record of your journey towards your goal. The detailed monitoring chart—

called simply "The Chart"—in Chapter 6 offers a good way to conduct self-monitoring. (The smaller version below is for illustrative purposes only.) The Chart can be used to track any behavior, including eating, exercising, smoking, sleeping, watching television, and taking medication. Not only will self-monitoring help you keep track of what you are doing, it can also have a positive impact on the goal you are trying to achieve. In fact, charting your behavior is what we call a "psychological freebie." It may seem trivial, something that doesn't take much time or effort, but it packs a powerful punch.

The Chart (See Chapter 6 for complete version.)

My desired health behavior is: _____.
(Be specific.)

I will practice this behavior _____ days per week.

My short-term goal is _____.

My long-term goal is _____.

SUN	MON	TUE	WED	THU	FRI	SAT

 Time and again, research has shown that the simple act of monitoring a behavior can change that behavior. We call this the *self-monitoring*

effect. Behaviors, such as exercise, are likely to increase when they are monitored, and behaviors, such as eating high-fat foods or smoking, are likely to decrease with monitoring.

Is monitoring the answer to all lifestyle changes? Does it come with a money-back guarantee? Sorry—there are no quick fixes here. Remember, monitoring is just one of the five SMART skills that will help you make changes in your behavior. Here's what's behind the "magic."

Monitoring your behavior does several things. First, it puts up a barrier to the tricks your mind can play. It creates a visual account of your actual behavior. If you have a blank spot on your chart because you didn't exercise, you will be forced to deal with it. Given this evidence, you will have to consider the reason why you didn't. The same thing goes for the amount of ice cream you ate. Was it a lot? Was it a little? Monitoring eliminates the uncertainty by turning "a lot" or "a little" into an actual measurable amount.

Monitoring is especially important during the early stages of a behavior change because it allows you to stay aware of where you are and recognize problems early on.

Monitoring also provides a visual reminder, or cue, for you to practice the behavior. However, your monitoring chart will serve as a visual reminder only if it is kept in a place where you can easily see it. If you place your chart in a desk drawer, it will not have the same effect as placing it in a highly visible location, such as on the refrigerator, the bathroom mirror, or the back of your front door. When you place your chart where you can see it without effort, you are changing your environment in a way that will increase your chances of engaging in the desired behavior.

Finally, the monitoring chart serves as a visual reinforcement or reward (see "Treat Yourself" on page 57). By watching your progress on the chart, you will be more likely to continue the behavior.

A rrange Your World for Success

Arranging your world for success is surprisingly simple, yet it can have immediate positive effects on your behavior. For example, at a recent dinner with colleagues and friends, the topic turned to unhealthy habits. One dinner guest described her habit of adding extra salt to her food and asked for help with decreasing her salt intake. As the token psychologists at the table, we told her we would help her decrease the chance of ingesting additional salt with her meal right at that moment. All the other guests were waiting for some sort of hocus-pocus.

Instead, we scanned the dinner table (evaluated her environment). We noticed the salt shaker was within arm's length of the woman, so we simply moved it to the opposite end of the table. We proclaimed with great satisfaction that this gesture had significantly decreased her chances of using excess salt during the meal. Everyone thought this was silly, but guess what? The woman did not use extra salt for the rest of the meal, even though she said she normally would have. The point is that changing your environment can have immediate and powerful effects on your behavior.

Arranging the world around you means doing things that will increase the odds of your being successful. No one can be successful 100 percent of the time. Life will always throw challenges and barriers your way. You may be going along nicely with an exercise program and then get sick and be unable to exercise for a week. You may be sticking with a healthy diet and then the holidays roll around. You may have out-of-town guests to entertain. The weather might be bad, the car can break down, your boss can ask you to stay late at work, or the kids can get sick—the list goes on and on. There are some things you simply can't control. This is why we want you to take charge of the things you *can* change in order to succeed.

Changing your world means arranging your immediate surroundings to increase the chances of a healthy behavior, such as a proper diet or exercise, or to decrease the chance of an unhealthy behavior, such as smoking. If you want to eat low-fat foods but you have a pantry stuffed with cookies and chips, the chances of eating the low-fat foods are slim. However, if you want to eat low-fat foods and your pantry contains nothing but low-fat foods, you're much more likely to eat them. Unfortunately, many people fail to arrange their environments to promote positive change.

The challenge is to make your environment support your desired behavior so that it becomes automatic, but how do you do this? Try this simple exercise:

 If you want to exercise every morning, think about how to modify your environment to increase your chances of success. Go ahead and list your ideas:

Changes I Can Make to My Environment That Will Promote Morning Exercise

1. _____

2. _____

3. _____

4. _____

5. _____

6. _____

Here are some of the suggestions we came up with. You may have similar ideas, or you might have thought of others not on our list.

✔ Set the alarm clock to include the amount of time it takes to get ready + travel time + exercise time.
✔ Before going to bed, lay out your exercise clothes where you will see them immediately upon rising.
✔ The night before, prepare any food or drink you plan to have before exercising.
✔ Put sticky notes on your bathroom mirror and refrigerator reminding you to exercise.
✔ Inform others (family, friends, your dog) that you *will* (not that you plan to) exercise in the morning.

In an ideal world, someone would come to your bedroom each morning, wake you, dress you, feed you, take you to your exercise location, and exercise with you. Just think, what would be the chances of not exercising under these circumstances? Because most of us cannot afford this kind of assistance, we must try to get as close to it as possible. If you do the four items listed above, but still don't exercise, it will be due to either an emergency or illness, or because you choose not to.

Arranging your world for success is all about taking control of your life in small but powerful ways. If you can break down the small barriers, you will find that making and sticking with changes get easier and easier. List below a health behavior that you want to change *other than exercise*, such as eat healthy food, quit smoking, get more sleep, or remember to take your medication. Then, list the things you can do to set yourself up for success. As we're sure you'll see, with a little thought you can be successful in creating healthy changes.

Behavior I want to change: _____

Ways I can arrange my environment to support this change:

1. _____

2. _____

3. _____

4. _____

5. _____

6. _____

7. _____

ACTION TIP
Getting over Gym Phobia

Going to a gym or health club can be a little intimidating, so here are some tips to help you ease into the gym experience.

Find a gym or club that is close to your home or work—the closer, the more likely you are to go. Then take a tour and ask as many questions as you want before you join. Make sure it's the right gym for you. Take advantage of free personal training or use of a trainer for a short time; you'll get familiar with the equipment and develop a work-out routine. Finally, if you're feeling a little self-conscious, train at off-peak hours when the gym is less crowded.

Remember, every person in the gym was unsure of himself in the beginning. The longer you stick with it, the more comfortable it will become.

R ecruit a Support Team

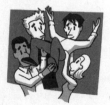 Ultimately, the changes you make to your lifestyle are your responsibility; they are under your control and will primarily benefit you. However, your family, friends, co-workers, and others can play a big role in your success.

The people in your life can be powerful motivators, strong reinforcers, and unfortunately sometimes the major barriers to making lifestyle changes. Family, friends, and co-workers are a part of your environment. As we discussed in the section on arranging your world for success, the people in your life can either facilitate lifestyle change or slow it down.

Knowing this, seek to maximize the positive influence of others. The key is to take charge and set up a team of supporters who will be encouraging and work with you. Most often, people leave the influence of those around them up to chance. They try to make changes on their own, and are either pleasantly surprised when friends and family offer encouragement and support, or frustrated when they seem uninterested or act as barriers to change. If you are going to make the effort to change your lifestyle and become healthier, why leave such a potentially powerful influence to chance? Let's take a look at what you can do to "rally the troops."

Think of those around you as an "army" of support. This may sound a bit self-centered. After all, you're not paying for their help the way you would professionals, such as trainers, coaches, or counselors. In reality, however, family, friends, co-workers, and even total strangers often are willing to help you make changes to improve your health without expecting anything in return. Why? We want to think that most people are just naturally eager to help one another.

If you think about this idea from a slightly more skeptical, yet scientific, perspective, it does make sense. Helping others can be a rewarding experience that is reinforced by the feelings it produces. For many people, knowing their actions have helped someone lose weight, stop smoking, become more physically fit, overcome an addiction, or reduce stress produces feelings of satisfaction, contentment, and even empowerment. Simply put, it just feels good to help others.

The people who agree to help you can be placed into two categories: change partners and supporters. Both are good, and both can help. Let's take a look at what each has to offer.

Change Partners

Change partners are people similar to you; they are also trying to make a lifestyle change. You can partner with them in your mutual endeavors. The advantage of being change partners is that both partners will have the satisfaction of helping someone else and the support they need for changing their own behaviors.

Supporters

Although supporters are not necessarily making changes themselves, they have agreed to support you and "be there" for you throughout the process. They may already have undergone the changes you are trying to make, or they may simply care about you enough to support your attempt to change your lifestyle.

Ideally, you will find a number of partners and supporters, but don't worry if you can't assemble an all-star team right away. Having a few dedicated people on your side is better than having either no one or a lot of people who aren't really committed to your goals. Now that you know other people can benefit from helping you, here is what you can do:

- ✔ Decide what kind of support will be most helpful
- ✔ See what kind of support is available
- ✔ Go out and get the support

Finding a Change Partner

Let's start with change partners. Where and how do you find them? Potential change partners are all around you— you simply haven't looked for them. A change partner can be your spouse or significant other, a friend, a parent, or another relative. Sometimes a potential partner will have already embarked on a lifestyle change and be struggling. In this case, the opportunity to get help and support (from you) will be most welcome. Other potential partners might be well on their way to making changes of their own and will share their experiences to bring you up to speed.

Consider your family and friends. Who among them is trying to change their lifestyle? Who is trying to exercise, diet, quit smoking, or make some other change? You probably never really looked at them as potential partners. Besides family, think about where you spend the majority of your time; who at your school or work is trying to make lifestyle changes? Does that person know you want to make a change, too? Again, we'd bet that you have never talked directly with this person and suggested a team approach. Becoming change partners can help both of you succeed. The following are places where you might consider looking for a partner:

✔ Home
✔ Work
✔ School
✔ Religious congregations
✔ Social gatherings (parks, bookstores, malls)
✔ Virtual communities (reputable health and fitness Web sites with chat rooms or partner programs)

Who would make a good change partner? Should you simply choose anyone making lifestyle changes who is willing to partner with you? Although you don't have to be too fussy, you should follow these general guidelines:

✔ Choose someone who is as committed to changing health behaviors as you are.
✔ Choose a partner who has similar, but not necessarily identical, goals.
✔ Choose a person whose daily schedule will allow him to work with you in making changes; for example, working out together, shopping for groceries together,

or talking to one another regularly about the progress you are both making.

 List three or more potential change partners. If you don't know their names, just describe them (for example, the woman you see walking in the park every morning).

1. _____

2. _____

3. _____

4. _____

5. _____

Finding a Supporter

Supporters are often easier to find than change partners, and you'll have a wider selection of people from which to choose, because they don't personally have to make lifestyle changes in order to qualify. Finding supporters also starts with looking at the people around you. Your immediate family and friends are important potential supporters. The difference between a supportive spouse or significant other and someone who has little interest in your lifestyle changes can really influence your success.

One of the best places to start looking for supporters is at home. Talk with the people closest to you. Be straightforward. Tell them about your goals, your concerns and fears, and why you need them to be there for you. Let them know that supporting you won't require a lot of effort on their part but that their support is critical to your success. Remember, most people want to be helpful, particularly when it doesn't require much effort. Supporters who live with you may be affected by your lifestyle changes more than those who don't. The changes you make in the foods you eat, the way you spend your time on a daily basis—such as going to the gym, walking in the park, going to bed earlier, practicing meditation, not going to bars, and not frequenting fast-food establishments—may have a significant effect on the people you're with the most. In that case, it can be extremely helpful to have supporters who are willing to become partners.

Having other people around you who are doing the things you want to *stop doing* will definitely create a challenge. Why? Think about the SMART skill: "Arrange Your World for Success." If you plan to stop eating high-fat foods, and your spouse, children, or the other people you live with keep these foods in abundance in the house, you are living in an environment that is less conducive to a low-fat diet. The same applies to things such as smoking, not exercising, excessive drinking, and poor sleep habits. Basically, if someone else is living an unhealthy lifestyle in your environment it will probably decrease your chances of success in making changes.

 Does this mean you will fail? No. Does it mean you will have more barriers to overcome? Yes.

Therefore, you may need to ask family and friends to make some changes in their own lifestyles in order to support you. Although everyone might not be willing, you may be pleasantly surprised to find that they will readily make the small changes you ask of them if they see the changes are beneficial. This might include not smoking around you, being a bit more flexible with daily schedules so you have time to exercise, or changing some of the social activities you participate in together.

Your success is one of the greatest rewards you can give your family and friends. If they see that their "sacrifices" are helping you become a healthier person, they are more likely to stick with you and the changes you have asked them to make. Let's put it this way: It's pretty hard to justify asking your family to give you time to exercise and not to eat junk food around you if they see you lying on the couch, watching television, and eating a big bag of chips!

Just how "healthy" do your supporters need to be? As a general rule, the more time you spend with a potential supporter on a daily basis, the more important it is for their health habits to be in line with your goals. If your Auntie Mae lives a thousand miles away but has agreed to talk with you any time you want or need to, she probably doesn't need to change her own eating or exercise habits in order to support you. However, your spouse, children, or co-workers, with whom you spend the majority of your time, will be a lot more helpful if their own lifestyle habits are in line with your goals.

The other advantage in having supporters whose lifestyles are consistent with your goals is that they are likely to be more sincere and enthusiastic in their support. It's more difficult for someone who eats poorly, doesn't exercise, and smokes to say with sincerity that they believe in the changes you are trying to make and understand their importance. This doesn't mean that someone with poor lifestyle habits isn't capable of caring about you and the changes you are trying to make; it simply means they may be less committed to your goals.

ACTION TIP
Stop Nagging

It's frustrating. You try to eat a low-fat diet and exercise, but your spouse isn't motivated to do the same. When it comes to changing health habits, spouses don't always see eye to eye. Although encouraging a spouse or loved one to take the steps they need for better health is important, encouragement alone may not always work. Instead, help your spouse by asking specific "action questions."

Start by asking what you can do to help your spouse to make the desired changes. You can also ask if more information would be helpful, such as figuring out which diet or exercise program would be most effective. If your spouse knows what to do, ask if you can help to create a plan for getting started. Encouragement is important, but action questions can really get the ball rolling.

In general, a supporter should be a person who:

✔ Cares about your health and well being
✔ Is willing to make small sacrifices to help you achieve your goals
✔ You spend a significant amount of time with on a daily basis
✔ You respect and care about

List three or more people who could be your supporters.

1. _____

2. _____

3. _____

4. _____

5. _____

Can I Go It Alone?

If recruiting a support team doesn't appeal to you, you may be wondering whether you can make lifestyle changes on your own. Remember, the SMART skills described in this book are designed to help you be successful in changing your lifestyle. The more of these skills you can use, the greater your chances at success. This doesn't mean you will fail if you don't have a support team. Many people have been able to make lifestyle changes without support. However, years of research show that the right kind of support is helpful. Don't give up if you can't rally a team, and don't spend the next 6 months waiting to start changing your behavior until you find the perfect team. Spend a few weeks looking for people who can work with you. Then, whether you have assembled a team or not, use the other skills you have learned and move forward.

Continue to look for partners and supporters as you embark on your lifestyle changes. You may find that friends, family, and co-workers will notice and encourage you. You may also find it easier to approach people and request their support. Finally, you will probably start to encounter people who are potential partners or supporters as you discover new places associated with your lifestyle changes; for example, parks, workout facilities, new restaurants, new Web sites, even new sections of the grocery store. Finding the right support team may take some time, so start making lifestyle changes and search for team members along the way.

T reat Yourself

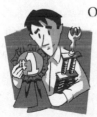 One of the most basic principles of behavioral science is that rewarded behaviors are more likely to be repeated. This principle is referred to as *reinforcement*, and it affects everyone—pets, children, and adults.

Understanding how reinforcement works will help you harness its power to make changes in your behavior.

Positive reinforcement occurs when a behavior is followed by an event that increases the chances that the behavior will be repeated. This process can take many forms. For example, positive reinforcement could include receiving money for a job well done, getting a compliment from a friend after you've lost weight, or giving your child a treat for being good. In each case, the chance of the particular behavior (doing a good job, losing weight, and being "good") being repeated is likely to be improved because it is associated with a pleasant event. Positive reinforcement is a great strategy for creating new behaviors.

With *negative reinforcement*, the chance that a behavior will be repeated is increased by removing something that is unpleasant. For example, if you have a headache and find that you can escape this unpleasant feeling by taking an aspirin, the behavior of taking the aspirin is likely to be repeated the next time you have a headache.

Keep in mind that the terms "positive" and "negative" don't necessarily refer to "good" and "bad." Negative reinforcement is not the same thing as punishment. If used properly, both types of reinforcement can help you continue performing your desired behaviors.

Reinforcement can take a variety of forms. All kinds of treats—money, candy, verbal praise, applause, or gold stars on a monitoring chart—can increase your chance of repeating a desired behavior. What works best? That's the tricky part, and it's an individual thing. What might be a powerful treat for one person might not be for someone else.

Chances are you already know what kinds of rewards are likely to increase your chances of success in changing your behavior. Here are some broad categories. Circle the ones that work for you.

✔ Monetary rewards (cash)
✔ Non-monetary gifts (clothes, music CDs)
✔ Social rewards (praise from friends and family)
✔ Activity rewards (going out to a movie or getting a manicure)
✔ Physiological rewards (pleasant sights, sounds, tastes, and smells)
✔ Psychological rewards (feelings of happiness, contentment, and satisfaction)

Why do we get into so much trouble with sweets, salty snacks, and other junk food? Food has the potential to be a powerful physiologic and psychological reward—it's a reinforcer that satisfies both our bodies and our minds. As an example, think about eating ice cream, which has a built-in reward system for most people. You purchase the ice cream and put some in your mouth. It's cool, refreshing, sweet, and creamy. Your taste buds come alive, and your visual, olfactory, and gustatory senses are stimulated. You smile. You're happy. Thus your ice cream eating behavior has been rewarded. What happens next? You take another bite, and another, and every bite you take gives you both physiologic and psychological rewards.

Once you have figured out what rewards are important for you, when should you give them to yourself? Again, we know from behavioral science that a new behavior needs to be rewarded frequently in order for it to become a permanent habit.

Developing a new habit means rewarding the new behavior over and over again until it becomes a normal part of your routine. Once it becomes a habit, you can back off the rewards a bit. Over time, you may find that the behavior itself has rewarding properties; for example, feelings of accomplishment and satisfaction. This frees you from having to reward the behavior over and over. However, ongoing occasional rewards will keep the new behavior going strong.

ACTION TIP
Effective Treats

✔ Decide on the reward before you start to make changes in your behavior.

✔ Determine when and how often you will treat yourself.

✔ Include your rewards on your monitoring chart and post it where you'll see it every day.

✔ Make sure that your rewards occur frequently in the beginning. For example, don't spend a month exercising before you get a reward. Small, frequent treats, such as a brief chat with a friend on the phone or taking the time to watch the sunset, are especially important in the beginning.

Treat Yourself Checklist Exercise

Fill in the blanks to create your reward schedule:

I will give myself _____ (reward) as a treat for
_____ (health behavior).

I will give myself _____ (reward) on the following
schedule: _____ _____
(how often you will give yourself the reward).

In addition to giving myself _____ (reward), if I
complete _____ (number of days, weeks, or months) of
_____ (health behavior), I will give myself a
bonus treat of _____
(choose a bonus reward).

Remember, a behavior that is rewarded, or
"treated," is likely to be repeated. If you reward
your exercise, diet, and non-smoking behaviors, over time you will find that these healthy behaviors have become rewarding on their own, and the need for
continued treats will slowly fade.

5

Stay on Track—Avoid Behavioral Drift

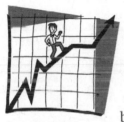 Now that you have learned the SMART skills, you can use them in combination with information and motivation to be successful in making lasting lifestyle changes. However, success does not mean being perfect. No matter how dedicated and committed you are, there will be periodic setbacks, but why?

First, life throws up all kinds of barriers to change—illness, injury, vacation, and work and home responsibilities. We interact with an environment that is constantly changing. Second, you are basically taking old behaviors and replacing them with new ones. The key word here is "new." The behaviors are not yet learned habits, and you will have a tendency to slip back into your old patterns.

Behavioral Drift

 The scientific term for this is *behavioral drift*, and it refers to the tendency to go back to old behavioral patterns when you are first making changes.

Everyone is affected by drift. We are all creatures of habit—and habits are strong, powerful things. When you begin to make changes in your lifestyle, there will be a strong pull toward your old habits. Behavioral drift affects everyone all the time. It's incredibly common, yet many people wonder why they seem to shift gradually back to their old ways just when they think they are doing a good at job at changing them. Behavioral drift always seems to sneak up on people, grab them, and pull them back to their old ways. No one ever warns us about behavioral drift. Well, consider this a warning.

Don't worry, though. Knowing that the dreaded drift exists is the most important part of preventing it. Now, let's discuss how to deal with it.

Don't Let the Drift Catch You

Now that you have read up to this point, you have every-thing you need to deal with the dreaded behavioral drift. Nothing in this section is new, except for an understanding of the drift itself. Here's a quick preview of how the skills you've learned can help:

✔ Monitoring your progress and using the other SMART skills will help you recognize the early stages of drift.
✔ Your understanding of motivation, rewards, and environmental barriers will enable you to find the cause of the drift.
✔ Your ability to recruit a support team and set achievable goals will help you modify any drift that does occur.

You see, once you have the tools to defeat it, the drift process is not quite so scary.

Dealing with behavioral drift involves three key actions:

1. Anticipating the causes of the drift
2. Having a plan to deal with the drift
3. Catching the drift in its earliest stages

ACTION TIP
Navigating the Grocery Aisles

Shopping for groceries can be tough when you're trying to eat healthy. How do you resist buying the high-calorie items that are not good for you? You're going to face temptations, but these simple tips will help:

- ✔ Write out your grocery list ahead of time. Not having a list puts you at risk of straying from a healthy diet. Check off each item as you shop.
- ✔ Avoid going up and down each aisle. Use your list to navigate past the cookies, chips, and other tempting items.
- ✔ Go shopping with a buddy, so you can focus on conversation rather than temptation.
- ✔ Reward yourself for sticking with your grocery list by purchasing one small treat for yourself.

Anticipating the Causes of the Drift

You have already done the most important part—you have learned that behavioral drift can and will occur. Now, make a list of the situations that are likely to cause you to backslide from your new health-related behaviors. This "What If" list will help you target situations that are likely to lead to behavioral drift. The details of this list will be different for each behavior, but the process and general topics are the same. Here are some common examples.

- ✔ What if the weather is bad and I can't exercise outside?
- ✔ What if we go out to dinner and they don't have the foods on my diet?
- ✔ What if we are traveling and I can't get to bed at a reasonable hour?
- ✔ What if I go to a bar and someone offers me a cigarette?
- ✔ What if my schedule changes and I can't do my relaxation exercises in the morning before work?
- ✔ What if my motivation levels decrease?
- ✔ What if the rewards I am using no longer work?
- ✔ What if I am sick or injured and unable to exercise, prepare certain meals, or take my scheduled medications?
- ✔ What if my change partner is no longer available?
- ✔ What if my supporters are no longer available?

 List three or more "What If" scenarios that might affect your success in achieving your health goals.

1. _____

2. _____

3. _____

4. _____

These situations will not necessarily cause behavioral drift, but they are good warning signs. Therefore, the longer the list is, the better. Leave no stone unturned. If you can anticipate it, you can plan for it—and if you can plan for it, you will know how to deal with it.

A Plan for Getting Back on Track

1. Answering the "What Ifs"

To develop your plan for dealing with drift, you need to come up with one or more answers for each of your "What If" questions. These situations do not guarantee drift will occur, but if it does, you will be able to remedy the problem. Similarly, if you find yourself drifting back into your old habits, you can use the "What If" list to figure out why. Here are some possible answers to "What If" questions:

What if I can't exercise outdoors because the weather is bad?
I can walk indoors at the local mall, or I can walk in place while watching television.

What if I can't do my normal exercise routine because I will be out of town?
I can call ahead and see if there are similar workout facilities where I will be staying, or I can walk inside or outside for 15 minutes.

What if my motivation level seems to be slipping?
I can challenge myself by answering the following questions honestly:

✔ What are the benefits of this new behavior?
✔ How important is it to improve my health?
✔ What am I doing right now instead of the new behavior? Are the reasons for doing it more important than bettering my health?

2. Your Drift Partner

In addition to answering the "What Ifs," your supporters can help you prevent the drift. Designate one person on your support team to be your drift partner. Ask this person's permission to call and talk when you first begin to drift. Your drift partner will encourage you to get back on track and remind you of your goals.

3. The Three-Day Rule

Now that you're armed with a plan for dealing with situations that can cause drift, you are ready to set up your "Drift Radar." Actually, you already have—your monitoring chart is the best way to alert you when you begin to drift. The rule of thumb for catching drift is to let the monitoring chart speak for itself. Don't guess at whether or not, and to what extent, you have done a new behavior; the monitoring chart will serve as your radar screen. By marking down your new health-related behaviors (exercise, dietary intake, taking medication regularly, or number of days of non-smoking), you will know whether or not you have practiced your target behavior. If the behavior seems to slip off the radar screen for a period of time, a red flag should be raised, and you will need to look at your "What If" list to see what's going on and what needs to be done.

 As a general guideline, you may be starting to drift if you have gone more than 3 days without practicing your new behavior. There may be good reasons why you haven't practiced the behavior, but that is not the point. In the early stages of lifestyle change, every day that a new behavior isn't practiced is another lost day of habit development. Even if you have good reasons for failing to practice your new behavior, simply not doing it will contribute to the drift. Look at your monitoring chart every day and be prepared.

Putting Everything into Perspective

Finally, put all of this information into perspective. If your goal is to eat a healthier diet, exercise regularly, practice relaxation exercises, get adequate sleep, or wear your seat belt every time you drive for the rest of your life, then missing 2–5 days of your new behavior is not the end of the world. The critical point is that you need to catch behavioral drift early, implement your plan, and get back on track. If you don't take the time to deal with drift, 2–5 days may turn into 2–5 weeks, months, or years. Anticipating the drift, knowing what situations can cause it, and having a plan to deal with it will keep you on the right track.

Ultimately it comes down to this: You are in control of your health, and you have the tools and techniques to make lifestyle changes. This is not magic. It's not a mystery. You can change any health-related behavior you want to and ultimately become a healthier person.

ACTION TIP
Get Control over Negative Thoughts

You try so hard to lose weight, exercise, or quit smoking. Then you have a setback, and with it come guilt and self-doubt. The trick is to control these negative thoughts so you don't give up. When you have a setback, take a minute and write down any negative thoughts you may have, such as: "I have no self-control" or "I don't have enough willpower." Now read your list aloud. Most negative thoughts aren't completely accurate, which reading aloud tends to demonstrate. Next, make a list of the times when you have shown self-control and willpower, and then read this list aloud. This little exercise will help you control negative thoughts and reach your health goals.

6

The Chart: Your All-in-One Behavior Change Tool

The Chart
The What, The Want, and The How

My health behavior is: _____ (be specific)

I will practice my behavior _____ days per week.

My short-term goal is _____.

My long-term goal is _____.

I will give myself _____(treat)

on the following schedule:

_____ (how often).

In addition to giving myself _____, when I

complete _____ (number of days, weeks, or months),

I will give myself a bonus treat of _____.

SUN	MON	TUE	WED	THU	FRI	SAT

Everything you have read so far can be condensed into this monitoring chart, which can be used to track healthy changes. The only catch is that you must first have a general understanding of the previous material. Once you understand the three necessary components: The What, The Want, and The How, this chart will help you make the desired changes.

We call this tool simply "The Chart," because on one level that is all that it is, a piece of paper. However, The Chart is also a lifestyle-change tool that contains all of the essential components for changing behavior.

The What

The Chart shows you what to do on a daily basis, how much you are supposed to do, and how frequently you should do it.

The Want

The Chart allows you to see your lifestyle change achievements on a daily, weekly, and monthly basis. Seeing your progress in black and white is a terrific reminder of your success. Success feels good, and feeling good strengthens your motivation.

The How

The Chart helps you accomplish all of the SMART behavior change skills discussed in this book. Here's how:

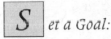 *et a Goal:*

The Chart allows you to specify your target behaviors.

 onitor Your Progresss:

The Chart allows you to keep track of your health-related behaviors and the progress toward your goal.

 rrange Your World for Success:

The Chart is a visual reminder that will cue you to practice health-related behaviors.

 ecruit a Support Team:

The Chart allows you to show others your specific goals and the work you have done so far.

T *reat Yourself:*

If you use visual rewards, such as gold stars or points, The Chart itself becomes the reward. It also allows you to see the rewards you will give yourself after you have practiced healthy behaviors.

This simple piece of paper can be of tremendous help when you are trying to make lifestyle changes. Making a chart can be as simple as grabbing a calendar and writing down your target behaviors, short- and long-term goals, and rewards. You can get more elaborate and design a chart on your computer, but more complicated charts are not necessarily better. In fact, the real key to The Chart's helpfulness and usefulness is your ability to look at it every day without any effort. A simple calendar posted on your refrigerator will be much more effective than a complex, custom-designed chart that sits in a drawer or in a stack of papers. So keep your chart simple, and put it on your refrigerator door today. Think of The Chart as your secret weapon. No one would ever suspect that such a simple thing could give you the edge in making successful lifestyle changes.

You can download a copy of The Chart from our website, www.livingsmart.diamedicapub.com.

PART II

Your Game Plan

*Y*ou now have all the ingredients to make *any* change in *any* health habit you want. That's a pretty powerful concept, but one that can also be a bit overwhelming. The following chapters will help you put the ideas in this book into specific actions.

This section contains specific *game plans* for change. We've chosen four issues that many people struggle with: sticking with a diet or exercise program, getting better sleep, and remembering to take medication. These game plans offer unique tips that are suited for these particular health behaviors, and they can help you jump start your progress. Of course, the game plans can be used to change any other behavior, too.

7

My Diet Game Plan

The What—Important Information about Your Diet

The average American's diet is not great. Just take a look at these figures from a study published in the *Journal of Food Composition and Analysis*:

✔ Sweets and desserts, soft drinks, and alcoholic beverages make up almost 25 percent of all calories consumed by Americans.

✔ Salty snacks and fruit-flavored drinks comprise 5 percent of the calories consumed by Americans.

✔ Healthy foods, such as vegetables and fruit, make up only 10 percent of the caloric intake in the U.S. diet.

✔ A large proportion of Americans are undernourished in terms of vitamins and minerals, even though they eat a lot of food.

 A key conclusion from this study is that people shouldn't necessarily be eating less, they should be eating differently. Here are some simple tips from the U.S. Department of Health and Human Services and the U.S. Department of Agriculture. (For more information see: http://www.mypyramid.gov/pyramid/grains_tips.html.)

✔ A healthy diet should emphasize fruits, vegetables, whole grains, and fat-free or low-fat milk and milk products. It should include lean meats, poultry, fish, beans, eggs, and nuts, and it should be low in saturated fats, trans fats, cholesterol, salt (sodium), and added sugars.

✔ Try to eat a variety of whole fruits rather than fruit juice. Eat vegetables of every color, including dark green vegetables (broccoli, kale, and other dark leafy greens), orange vegetables (carrots, sweet potatoes, pumpkin, and winter squash), and beans and peas (pinto beans, kidney beans, black beans, garbanzo beans, split peas, and lentils).

✔ Eat foods that are rich in calcium every day, including low-fat or fat-free milk, or an equivalent amount of low-fat yogurt and/or low-fat cheese (1½ ounces of cheese equals 1 cup of milk). If you don't or can't consume milk, eat lactose-free milk products and/or calcium-fortified foods and beverages.

✔ Eat at least 3 ounces of whole-grain cereals, breads, crackers, rice, or pasta every day. Make sure that grains such as wheat, rice, oats, or corn are referred to as "whole" in the list of ingredients.

✔ Eat lean protein. Make sure your meats are broiled, baked, or grilled, and include fish, beans, peas, nuts, and seeds in your sources of protein.

ACTION TIP
Control Your Snacking Habits

Are you a snacker? Snacking is a habit for many people. It has little to do with hunger, and can keep you from reaching your health goals. Here are some tips to help you curb your snacking habit:

- ✔ Keep a food diary for 1 week. As you record what you eat, write down what you were doing at the time and whether or not you were actually hungry. This will help you identify your snacking pattern. For example, you may tend to snack while watching television.
- ✔ Next, to help you deal with situations where you tend to snack, substitute other activities that make it hard to snack. Try playing with your kids or pets, or exercise while you watch television. Knowing your snacking patterns and having actions to prevent them will help improve your eating habits.

The Want—Are You Motivated to Change Your Eating Habits?

This is the time to be honest about what you *really* want to do about your eating habits. The simple question is: Are you motivated to change? If your answer to this question is "no," you will not be able to change your eating behavior, and this is probably not a good time for you to try to do something about your diet. You may want to change your eating habits at another time. The principles and SMART skills outlined in this book will still be available when you become motivated to change.

If your answer to this question is "yes"—great! You understand that some degree of motivation is necessary to change behavior and to keep it going over the long term. You have to *want* to make changes in your eating in order to be successful.

Let's examine more closely the degree to which you're motivated to change your eating habits. Rate your level of motivation on the scale below.

1	2	3	4	5	6	7	8	9	10
A little									Completely
motivated									motivated

If your degree of motivation is less than 3, go back to Chapter 3 and use the motivation-boosting strategies. It's important to find your own reasons for changing your eating patterns. Eating a healthy diet needs to be important to you personally in order for you to be motivated to change.

If you rated your motivation as 4 or greater, you're ready to get started. Remember, you don't have to be a "10"—completely motivated. If you rate yourself at mid-point on the scale, you still have enough motivation to start changing your eating habits. As we've said before, motivation typically comes and goes over time. Whenever you feel your motivation level decreasing, go back and use the boosters.

The How—SMART Skills That Can Change Your Eating Habits

SMART skills are the key to changing habits and routines. You read about them earlier, but now let's make them specific to eating. Read through the examples below to see what you can use to help you start your new habits.

S et a Goal

Goals for improving eating habits are as numerous and individual as the people who want to change their diets. However, some eating goals pop up more frequently than others, and they have several common themes. We often get comments such as: "I want to consume fewer calories," "My goal is to eat less fast food," or "My goal is to cut sweets and desserts out of my diet."

These are great ideas, but they are too general. Remember, setting a goal requires you to be specific—the more specific, observable, and measurable the goal, the more likely you are to succeed. You need to identify a behavior that is observable and that can be measured. You need to be sure that it is a goal you can achieve—don't set yourself up for failure. How could you make the goal, "I want to consume fewer calories" specific, observable, and measurable?

 Write your answers below:

General goal: "I want to consume fewer calories"

Make it specific: _____

How could you observe it? _____

How could you measure it? _____

_____

We came up with a more specific goal of "eat 1,900 calories per day." This is observable, because you can see yourself putting portions containing a certain number of calories into your mouth. Also, calories can be counted or measured. Calorie content can be found in books or on the Internet, and labels on most foods identify the number of calories in a serving (be sure to double check the number of servings in a package or a container—often there are more than one).

How can you make the general goal, "I want to eat less fast food," specific, observable, and measurable?

Make it specific: _____

_____

How could you observe it? _____

_____

How could you measure it? _____

_____

M onitor Your Progress

Monitoring what you eat and reducing your caloric intake may take a bit of effort, depending on the goal you've set. It's important to keep track of the calories in *everything* you eat

ACTION TIP
Managing Fast Food Temptations

In today's fast-paced lifestyle, fast food is a major convenience. But it can quickly become a very unhealthy habit. If you're on a diet, you know how hard it is to resist visiting your favorite fast food restaurants. If fast food is your weakness, try these tips:

✔ Bring your lunch to work, and plan dinners at home so you aren't tempted to eat out.

✔ If your favorite fast food restaurant is on your daily commute, change your route or place a sticky note on your dashboard that says "No Fast Food."

✔ Avoid getting fast food for your kids. Your family will benefit from healthier meals.

✔ Choose a special reward for you and your family for each day you skip fast food.

Before you know it, fast food will become less tempting, and you'll reach your health goals more quickly.

and drink during the day. You need to keep your monitoring chart close by, because you probably eat at home, work, and in restaurants or fast food places. Some people use a handheld computer for this purpose. If you prefer, you can make several copies of the monitoring chart (see Chapter 6), and keep them in your pocket, briefcase, or handbag. Just make sure that whatever you use is always within easy reach. You don't want to rely on your memory.

Keeping track of fast foods and desserts may be somewhat easier. If you set a goal of limiting fast food meals to one per week, you could use your monitoring chart to keep track of this behavior. Be sure to post the chart in a visible place, so you are reminded of your goal and your weekly progress. Similarly, if you are trying to decrease the number of desserts and sugary snacks in your diet, the monitoring chart or a calendar on the wall will work perfectly.

A rrange Your World for Success

This SMART skill can be incredibly powerful in helping you meet your eating goals. The idea is to set up the world around you so that you are successful in changing your eating habits. If you don't have high-calorie foods in your environment, you won't be able to eat them. If you don't bring fast food into your world, you won't eat it. These strategies make perfect sense when you think about making the world around you support your efforts for successful eating.

- ✔ Remove all high-calorie foods from your kitchen and pantry.
- ✔ If you want special snacks for your children, keep them in a place where you can't see them, and keep them out of easy reach.
- ✔ "Arranging" begins at the grocery store. Only bring home food that will help you meet your goals.

✔ Have healthy snacks visible and readily available so you can get to them easily if you feel tempted to eat a high-calorie food.

✔ Post a reminder to yourself on the refrigerator door about your eating goals. Your monitoring chart could serve this purpose.

✔ Pack a healthy lunch the night before so that it's ready to take to work with you in the morning.

R ecruit a Support Team

Research clearly shows that this SMART skill is critical—having support will definitely help you stick with any diet and successfully change your eating habits. The problem is that not everyone is likely to be aware of your goal, so you may not automatically get the support you need. Tell people you are making changes in your eating habits, but also tell them exactly what they can do to help you. Here are some simple, useful strategies for getting support:

✔ Let your family and friends know you are trying to change your eating habits and stick with a healthier diet.

✔ Talk with them about how challenging this is for you, and let them know their help is critical for your success.

There are many ways other people can support your efforts, some of which may be more practical and feasible than others:

✔ Ask them if they would like to join you in changing eating habits.

✔ Ask them to periodically give you verbal encouragement and praise for sticking with your plan.

✔ Ask them to call and leave encouraging voice mail messages.

✔ Ask if they will send you supportive e-mails or text messages.

✔ Let your spouse or significant other know what help you need to stick with your diet, such as not eating dessert in front of you or not offering you junk food.

T reat Yourself

A diet or any other change in your eating habits that is painful simply will not work. You need some ongoing benefit or reward from your diet to keep up your motivation. What can you do? If your goal is to lose 20 pounds by eating a healthier diet, and the reward is the lost weight, you are simply setting yourself up for failure. Why? You will fail because you will not lose 20 pounds in the first week—you may not even lose 2 pounds!

What will keep you going? What treat or reward will get you through the first week of the diet and on to the second? How will you treat yourself after week two so you can continue on to week three? If you build treats into your diet on a weekly basis, you will be more likely to stick with it and ultimately reach your goal. Does treating yourself mean a banana split or a pizza at the end of the week? Probably not. Here are some ideas about how you might treat yourself on a weekly basis:

✔ Designate a specific reward that you will give yourself at the end of each week that you stick with your diet. For example, you might treat yourself with a low-fat ice cream cone at the end of week one, a movie with a friend at the end of week two, shopping for a new outfit at the end of week three, and so on. Write down each treat on your calendar or monitoring chart so you will be reminded of it often.

✔ Alternatively, you can give yourself a "cheat night" once a week if you stick with your diet. On your cheat night (and *only* on your cheat night), you can eat whatever you like. You'll probably find that early on you will really splurge, but over time your "cheating" will become less and less frequent.

✔ Finally, a really simple strategy you can use in addition to the ones above is to place gold stars on your monitoring chart for each day you stick with your diet. This may sound silly, but the act of putting the stars on the chart will remind you of your progress and help you keep eating healthy food.

You now have a game plan for sticking with any diet. You have everything you need to succeed. It's time to look forward and envision yourself as a healthier and happier individual. Applying this game plan means you have begun to take control of your health destiny.

8

My Exercise Game Plan

The What—Important Information about Your Exercise Program

We have said many times that there is no magic pill, but when it comes to being healthy, physical activity along with a healthy diet is the closest we can get. Let's review some facts from *Physical Activity: The Magic Pill*, a booklet published by The President's Council on Fitness and Sports:

✔ Moderate physical activity helps lower cholesterol, blood sugar, and blood pressure.

✔ Exercise strengthens muscles and improves flexibility and range of motion, thereby protecting the joints against osteoporosis. It also relieves the symptoms of arthritis.

✔ Physical exercise reduces your risk of cardiovascular disease, stroke, and certain kinds of cancer. It also helps reduce the symptoms of anxiety and depression.

✔ Walking 15 minutes at a moderate rate will burn approximately 100 calories; thus, 5 days of walking burns 500 calories. Since there are approximately 3,000 calories in a pound, a 5-day-per-week walking program can reduce your weight by 1 pound every 6 weeks, assuming that you don't increase your caloric intake.

We often hear about "moderate" levels of activity, but it can be difficult to figure out exactly what this means. Here are some examples of light, moderate, and heavy physical activity:

Sedentary	Light
Watching television	Slow walking
Reading	Cooking food
Eating	Washing dishes
Typing on the computer	Putting away groceries
Talking on the phone	Child care
Standing in line	Croquet
Riding in a car	Mild stretching
General office work	Billiards

Moderate	Vigorous
Brisk walking	Walking up stairs
Weight lifting	Jogging/running
Tai chi	Bicycling (faster than 12 mph)
Golf	Swimming
Cleaning house	Cross-country skiing
Gardening	Singles tennis
Playing softball	Jumping rope
	Playing basketball

For more detailed information, and to read the entire booklet, go to the President's Council on Fitness and Sports Web page at: www.fitness.gov.

Action Tip
Get the Ball Rolling

We all know we need to exercise regularly, but it can be so hard to get started.

✔ You need a specific goal—saying you're going to exercise is not specific enough.
✔ Walking for 30 minutes on Monday, Wednesday, and Friday from 5:00 to 5:30 P.M. is specific. The more specific the goal, the more likely you are to succeed.
✔ Be realistic. Don't set goals that are too big and therefore unattainable. Pick reasonable goals that you can reach. Start small, be successful, and gradually build, and you'll be on your way in developing any healthy habit.

The Want—Are You Motivated to Exercise?

It's time to focus on exercise and be honest. Do you to *want* to make changes in your exercise program in order to be successful? Are you motivated to change your exercise level—whether this means starting to exercise or increasing the amount of exercise you do? If your answer is "no," you won't be able to make lasting changes in your exercise behaviors, and this isn't a good time to begin a new program.

If your answer to this question is "yes"—great! You have some degree of motivation to change your behavior and keep it going over the long term. Let's examine more closely the degree to which you're motivated to change your exercise levels. Rate your level of motivation on this scale:

1   2   3   4   5   6   7   8   9   10
A little   Completely
motivated   motivated

If your degree of motivation is 3 or less, go back to Chapter 3 and use the motivation-boosting strategies. Exercise and physical activity need to be important to you personally in order for you to be motivated, so find your own reasons for exercising.

If you rated your motivation as 4 or higher, you're ready to get started. Remember, you don't have to be a "10"—completely motivated. Even if you rate yourself at midpoint on the scale, you have enough motivation to start your new exercise program. We've said it earlier, motivation typically comes and goes over time. Whenever you feel your motivation level getting low, go back and use the boosters.

The How—SMART Skills for Making Exercise Happen

You've got The What and The Want, but *how* do you make exercise a reality? Here are some specific examples of

SMART skills that focus on exercise. Read through them to learn about how to start your new exercise routine.

S et a Goal

There are endless possibilities when it comes to physical activity. As you might imagine, we couldn't even begin to think of all the possible exercise goals. However, most people seem to share some common objectives. We also find that the changes people want to make follow some general themes, such as "I want to do cardiovascular exercise every day," "I want to get stronger," or "I want to improve the way my body looks."

These are wonderful ideas, but they are far too general. As we have noted elsewhere, having a goal means identifying a specific behavior that can be changed. Your goal needs to be observable and measurable. The more specific, observable, and measurable the goal, the more likely you are to succeed. Your goal also needs to be one that you can achieve. How could you make the goal "I want to do cardiovascular exercise every day" specific, observable, and measurable? Write your answers below.

General goal: "I want to do cardiovascular exercise every day"

Make it specific: _____

_____

How could you observe it? _____

_____

How could you measure it? _____

_____

One specific exercise might be to walk on a treadmill for 30 minutes every day of the workweek, with weekends off. Cardiovascular exercise is not a specific behavior, but walking on a treadmill can be observed, and you can time how long you walk during each exercise session. Whether you walk on a treadmill or at a track, in the park or at the mall, walking is one of the simplest exercises you can do, but be sure to keep track of your time using a watch or stopwatch.

Should you start at 30 minutes right off the bat? Probably not. Remember, your goal is to reach a level where you are walking 5 days a week for 30 minutes. If you are just getting started, the most important thing you can do is to make sure you succeed. This is the concept of pacing, which we talked about earlier. Let's take another look at pacing.

If you think you can walk for 30 minutes, but aren't sure, what might happen? You will probably make it through the first day without much difficulty. What happens if you wake up the next morning and are sore and worn out? Your chances of walking again the second day go way down. You might skip the next walking session, and then you are off to a poor start toward your exercise goal.

In order to guarantee that each exercise session is a success, take the amount of exercise you *know* you can do and cut it in half for the first week. If you know you can do 30 minutes, walk for no more and no less than 15 minutes the first week. Each week, add 5 more minutes to the workout, no more and no less.

Your exercise time will look like this:

Week 1	15 minutes
Week 2	20 minutes
Week 3	25 minutes
Week 4	30 minutes

Once you have reached the 30-minute goal, you can add more time or walk more quickly. The most important concept here is that, in order to exercise regularly, you must develop the exercise habit *before* you will be able to develop your physical conditioning.

M onitor Your Progress

Monitoring your exercise is really quite simple and well worth the effort. You have a number of options. You can take your monitoring chart with you when you walk at a gym, and simply mark off the time you started walking and the time you finished. You can do the same thing on a PDA. You could also wait and fill in the monitoring chart at home at the end of each day. As you gradually increase your level of activity, note these changes on the chart. If you find it helpful, you can get "fancy" by graphing your progress. The American Heart Assoication (www.americanheart.org) and the President's Council on Fitness (www.fitness.gov) have several programs to help you track your progress. Finally, be sure to post the chart in a visible place to remind you of your goal and your weekly progress.

A rrange Your World for Success

This SMART skill will help you break down the barriers that keep you from exercising. We all know what they are: getting up late, forgetting where you put your workout clothes, not having enough time to exercise and still get to your job on time, bad weather, or an unexpected appointment. The barriers seem to jump out at you from every direction. By arranging your world ahead of time, you can head off these problems before they stop you from exercising. Here are a few suggestions that will help you break through some of the most common barriers to exercising.

✔ Designate specific times for exercising each day; for example, 6:30 A.M. and/or 5:30 P.M. If you are already going to the gym several times a week, at different times, you don't need a game plan—you're a gym rat like us.

✔ Mark the times you plan to exercise on your calendar, in your appointment book, or on your PDA.

✔ Have your exercise gear in your bag ready to go, or consider keeping your gear in a locker if one is available at your gym.

✔ If you exercise first thing in the morning, set your alarm clock to allow for the time it takes to get ready, travel, and exercise. Before you go to bed, lay out your exercise clothes where you will see them immediately upon rising. Prepare any food (such as a power bar or a piece of fruit) or drink you plan to have before exercising.

✔ Put post-it notes on your bathroom mirror and refrigerator reminding you to exercise.

✔ Inform others (family, friends, your dog) that you *will* exercise in the morning (not that you plan to).

R ecruit a Support Team

Working out with a partner makes exercise fun and adds accountability, so:

✔ Tell family, friends, and co-workers that you are starting an exercise program and ask if they will join you.

✔ Look for people at the park or gym who are exercising by themselves at the same time as you. They might be perfect partners. When you find exercise partners, make sure they are as committed to exercising as you are.

✔ Ask your family and friends to call and leave phone messages of encouragement.

✔ Tell your spouse or significant other you need help in sticking with it (for example, giving you time to exercise, watching the children, joining you in the workout).

T reat Yourself

Let's face it: Many people who start an exercise program do it because they need to improve their health, rather than because they see it as fun. Once you develop the exercise habit, you will enjoy it, look forward to it, and even crave it. But exercise may not be so rewarding when you first start. This makes it critical that you give yourself treats as an incentive to keep going. Here are a few suggestions:

✔ Enjoy a low-calorie snack after your workouts.
✔ Treat yourself to new workout shoes, apparel, or equipment, once you have stuck with it for a few weeks.
✔ If you don't always have enough time to relax after your workout, treat yourself to some time in the sauna, steam room, or Jacuzzi after exercising. Or, at least try to arrange an uninterrupted shower or bath at home.
✔ Give yourself a "cheat night" on your exercise plan when you stick with your workout schedule for a whole week.
✔ Put gold stars on your monitoring chart after each workout. As we've said before, this sounds silly, but it works.

 The particular treat you choose is not as important as making sure you schedule it for *after* you finish exercising. Building rewards into your routine will help your exercise program become a permanent habit. Once it has become a habit, you can slowly give up the rewards if you want to.

Exercise is a lifelong activity. Lifelong, however, doesn't mean every single day for the rest of your life. This game plan will provide you the specifics you need to get your exercise program up and running, and stick with it. If you miss some workouts, no problem. Just focus on exercising more days than not as your long-term goal.

Action Tip
For Mothers Only: Fit Exercise into Your Schedule

Mothers are some of the busiest people in the world, and their hectic schedules often leave little time for exercise. Here are three tips to help you fit exercise into your day.

✔ Examine your schedule hour by hour. You'll be surprised by how many gaps of 15–20 minutes you actually have to squeeze in some exercise.

✔ Next, do double duty. Walk around the soccer field while the kids are practicing, or walk or jog in the neighborhood where their piano lessons are taught.

✔ You probably have a friend or neighbor who is as busy as you are. Set up a "kid swap," where you each agree to watch each other's kids while the other exercises.

✔ Finally, ask your spouse or significant other to watch the kids while you exercise.

These strategies may not get you into the gym everyday, but they *will* help you become more active.

9

My Sleep Game Plan

The What—Important Information about Sleep

We all know what it feels like to not get a good night's sleep. Poor sleep is a nightly reality for many people. A 2005 poll by the National Sleep Foundation found that up to 75 percent of adult Americans reported sleep problems at least a few nights a week, up from 62 percent in 1999. The National Highway Traffic Safety Administration estimates that each year up to 100,000 police-reported accidents involve drowsiness.

Research clearly suggests that poor-quality sleep can put you at greater risk for diminished work productivity, anxiety and depression, and motor vehicle accidents, as well as increased risk for colon and breast cancer, heart disease, and diabetes. This means that improving your quality of sleep is a reasonable and important lifestyle goal.

The Want—Are You Motivated to Change Your Sleep Habits?

Most people who suffer from the effects of poor sleep really do want better quality sleep. However, getting a good night's sleep requires you to change some of your current habits. You will have to do things differently, and so we are back to this important question: Are you motivated to change your routines in a way that will result in better sleep? If your answer is "no," this is probably not a good time for you to try to do something to improve your sleep habits. The principles and the SMART skills will still be here when you find yourself motivated to change.

If your answer to this question is "yes"—great! You have The Want to make changes in your sleep habits in order to get better quality sleep.

Let's examine more closely the degree to which you're motivated to change your sleep-related routines. Rate your level of motivation on the scale below.

1   2   3   4   5   6   7   8   9   10
A little   Completely
motivated   motivated

If your degree of motivation is 3 or less, go back to Chapter 3 and use the motivation-boosting strategies. It's important to find your own reasons why better sleep is important.

If you rated your motivation as 4 or greater, you're ready to get started. As we've said before, you don't have to be a "10"—completely motivated. If you rate yourself at midpoint on the scale, you have enough motivation to start changing your sleep habits. Whenever you feel your motivation level decreasing, go back and complete the motivational exercises.

The How—SMART Skills for Improving Your Sleep

You know that sleep is important, and you want to improve the quality of your sleep by changing your sleep-related routines. Now that you've got The What and The Want, it's time to make The How a reality. The following specific examples of SMART skills focus on sleep. Read them to learn about how to start your new sleep routine.

S et a Goal

You may say you want better sleep. Seems straightforward enough, doesn't it? Let's stop for a minute and be more specific. What do you *really* want? Do you want to sleep more hours? Do you want to go to bed earlier? Get up earlier? Sleep longer on weekdays? Sleep longer on weekends? Go to bed and stay asleep all night? There are many possible goals. To make sure you reach your true sleep goal, you must be *specific* about what you want. Then you need to be specific about what behaviors you need to change in order to reach that goal. Everything must be measurable and observable. "Better sleep" is not measurable or observable. Goals such as sleeping through the night without waking up, sleeping for 8 hours, 5 nights a week, and going to bed at 9:30 P.M. are all specific, observable, and measurable actions. However, they are still a bit too general. How do you make the goal "sleep for 8 hours" as specific as possible? Give it a try below.

General goal: "I want to sleep for 8 hours."

Make it specific: _____

_____

How could you observe it? _____

_____

How could you measure it? _____

_____

Here's what we came up with:

✔ Get ready for bed at 8:00 P.M. by taking a warm bath.
✔ Wind down with a cup of decaffeinated tea.
✔ Read a book for 45 minutes.
✔ Go into the bedroom at approximately 9:15 P.M.
✔ Face the clock away from sight.
✔ Set the alarm for 5:45 A.M.
✔ Turn out the light.
✔ Allow 30 minutes to fall asleep.

These times and sleep routines may not fit exactly with your preferences, but the idea is to develop a detailed plan for what is necessary for you to reach your goal of sleeping for 8 hours.

M onitor Your Progress

Monitoring your sleep progress really translates into creating a sleep log, or diary. Whether it's a notebook, a calendar, or a handheld computer, make sure you monitor the following categories:

✔ The time you went to bed
✔ How sleepy you felt when you went to bed—use a 0–10 scale, with 0 being "not sleepy at all" and 10 being "extremely sleepy"
✔ In the morning, note the time you woke up (not what time you got out of bed)
✔ How refreshed/rested you felt—use the same 0–10 scale, with 0 being "not rested at all" and 10 being "extremely rested"
✔ How many times you remember waking up during the night and approximately how long you were awake

 Using these categories, your sleep log for one night might look something like this:

Sleep Monitoring Chart for Sunday/Monday
My goal is 8 Hours of Sleep Each Night
Wake Time Sunday_____
How refreshed (0–10)_____
Number of times woke up Sunday night _____
Bedtime Monday night _____
How Sleepy (0–10) _____

Continue to monitor your sleep progress, and you should see improvement within a week or so.

A rrange Your World for Success

Sleep is a behavior, and although it can be influenced by many medical conditions, the actions you take prior to sleeping will have a great impact on how well you sleep.

Here are some basic sleep guidelines:

✔ Go to bed and get up at a similar time every day. This may be more challenging on the weekends, but by using an alarm clock you can make sure your sleep cycle has a regular rhythm, which will help improve your sleep.

✔ Use your bed for only for sleeping. Don't use it for watching television, paying bills, or working. That way, when you go to bed, your body will know it's time to sleep.

✔ Reduce any noise in your room. If you can't reduce the noise, consider getting a "white noise" machine or foam ear plugs.

✔ Make sure your bed and bedroom are quiet and comfortable, and slightly cool. A hot room can disrupt sleep. A cool room and enough blankets to keep warm if needed are best.

✔ Set up a sleep routine you can follow every night. These are simply actions that you engage in to help you unwind. It's important to give your body cues that it's time to slow down and sleep. Try listening to relaxing music, read something soothing for 15 minutes, or practice meditation or prayer. Anything that calms you down and makes you drowsy is good. Be sure to practice the routine every night, regardless of how sleepy you are.

✔ Don't drink caffeine or alcohol, smoke, or exercise 4–6 hours before bedtime, because it can interfere with the quality of sleep

✔ Don't take naps. You want to be tired at bedtime. If you can't make it through the day without a nap, sleep less than 1 hour and take your nap before 3 P.M.

✔ Finally, if you can't fall asleep, don't stay in your bed for more than 20 minutes. Instead, get up, go into a dimly lit room and do something restful, such as listen to quiet music. Get back into bed when you feel sleepy.

R ecruit a Support Team

Recruiting a support team is critical if you sleep with another person, because your efforts to improve your sleep may significantly change your current sleep habits, and that, in turn, can affect the sleep of a spouse or significant other.

Communication with your sleep partner is essential. Before you make changes, talk to the person you live with. Let your partner know what your goal is, why you would want to make changes to your current routines, and why her help is important to your success. Be open to compromise. A 9:15 P.M. bedtime may be great for you, but it may not be for your sleep partner. Discuss how you can make it work for both of you. It may take your going to bed first and your significant other watching television in another room instead of the bedroom. Remember, if you want help and support, you need to be clear about what you want the other person to do, and be willing to compromise.

T reat Yourself

Getting a good night's sleep is one of those behaviors that is rewarding once it starts to happen. As we have all experienced, there is nothing better than feeling completely refreshed when you wake up. As you begin to develop better sleep habits and your sleep improves, you will feel rejuvenated and rewarded. However, there is nothing wrong with a little extra reward in the form of gold stars on your sleep log, or even a treat at the end of the week if your sleep is improving.

The better you sleep, the better you will feel. For most people, changing some of their routines is all that is needed to improve sleep. It may take some time, so give it a few weeks. Remember, sleep problems may be the sign of a more serious medical problem. Consult your doctor if changes in your routines don't seem to be helping.

10

My Medication Game Plan

The What—Important Information about Taking Medication

Did you know that 32 million Americans take three or more medications daily? It's estimated that 59 percent of them take their medication improperly. Whether it's taking too much, not enough, not completing a prescription, or not refilling a prescription, medication noncompliance has significant effects on health. Tens of thousands of deaths, numerous hospitalizations, and delayed recovery from illnesses occur each year because people don't take their medications properly.

Here are some statistics from the National Pharmaceutical Council, the American Hospital Association, and the American Heart Association:

✔ Medication noncompliance results in more than 125,000 deaths a year—twice as many people as are killed in motor vehicle accidents.

✔ People who regularly miss medication doses visit the doctor three times as much as those who take their medication as prescribed.

✔ Ten percent of all hospital admissions are the result of not taking prescription medications as prescribed.

✔ The average hospital stay due to medication noncompliance is 4.2 days.

✔ Twenty-three percent of all nursing home admissions are due to failure to take medications correctly.

Some of the most common errors people make when it comes to taking medication include:

✔ Forgetting to take medication
✔ Stopping before a medication is finished
✔ Taking the wrong dose
✔ Taking extra doses when a dose is missed
✔ Taking medication with the wrong food or drink
✔ Taking medication with other prescription or over-the-counter drugs, which can produce side effects
✔ Not filling or refilling a prescription

Taking medications as prescribed can be challenging, especially if you need to take them for a long period of time.

Taking medication daily is required for many conditions, including heart disease, high blood pressure, high cholesterol, some types of asthma, and HIV-AIDS. Taking medication on a regular basis is a behavior that can be developed into a habit, similar to changing your eating or exercise habits.

The Want—Am I Committed to Taking My Medication?

Most people say they are motivated to take a prescribed medication if it makes them feel better, improves their health, prevents an illness, or prolongs their lives. Are you motivated? Are you willing to make changes in your habits to make sure you will take your medication properly? Are you willing to endure the possible side effects of the medication, manage the costs associated with taking it, and deal with possible disruptions in your life that taking the medication may cause?

If your answer to this question is "yes"—great! You understand that some degree of motivation is necessary to change behavior and to keep it going over the long term, and you have The Want to make changes in your routines in order to be successful.

If your answer to this question is "no," you're not likely to succeed in changing your behavior in order to take your medication properly. It's time to figure out why taking your medication should be important. Below is one of the exercises from Chapter 3 that may help you decide whether taking medication on a regular basis is important to you, and why. Even if you completed this exercise earlier, try it again and focus specifically on the issue of taking medication.

Ask yourself these questions and write down the answers:

What behavior are you most likely to change as it relates to taking medications? _____

_____.

What made you select this particular behavior? _____

_____.

How would you feel if you were to make this change? ___

_____.

What else would be different about you? _____

_____.

What behavior have you been able to change in the past?

_____

_____.

Next, imagine yourself 5 years from now:

If my medication behavior stays the same, I will feel ____

_____.

If I keep doing exactly what I am doing now, I may experience

_____.

If I don't change a thing, my health will be _____

_____.

Imagine your loved ones 5 years from now:

If my medication behavior stays the same, it will affect my loved ones by _____

_____.

If my behavior stays the same, my loved ones may react by

_____

_____.

By taking the time to answer these questions, most people will be reminded of why they wanted to make changes in the first place. Simple as it seems, this little reminder can really boost your level of motivation. So, if you ever find your motivation slipping, repeat this exercise.

Now, let's examine more closely the degree to which you're motivated to stick with your medication regimen. Rate your level of motivation on the scale below.

1	2	3	4	5	6	7	8	9	10

A little   Completely
motivated   motivated

If your degree of motivation is 3 or less, go back to Chapter 3 and use the motivation-boosting strategies, including the one just given above. It's important to find your own reasons as to why you should take your medication as recommended.

If you rated your motivation as 4 or greater, you're ready to get started. Remember, you don't have to be a "10"—completely motivated. If you rate yourself at midpoint on the scale, you still have enough motivation to start changing your medication habits. As we talked about earlier, you can expect your motivation to come and go over time. Whenever you feel your motivation level decreasing, go back and use the booster exercises.

The How—SMART Skills for Taking Your Medication Consistently

Below are specific examples of SMART skills that focus on taking medication. Read through them to learn about how to stay on track with your medication regimen.

S et a Goal

Much like sleep, setting a goal for medication seems quite straightforward. "I want to take my medication properly" is a reasonable goal. However, as with all the behaviors we have already discussed, "taking my medication properly" is neither observable nor measurable. At this point you may be thinking: "Of course, I can take medication properly." Right? Not really. Taking medication properly involves developing a series of specific behaviors that are observable and measurable.

Try this exercise. How could you make the goal, "I want to take my medication properly" specific, observable, and measurable? Write your answers below.

General goal: "I want to take my medication properly."

Make it specific: _____

_____

How could you observe it? _____

_____

How could you measure it? _____

_____

While every medication regimen will differ, here are the specific behaviors we came up with that could define taking medication properly:

✔ Taking the right amount (number of pills)
✔ Taking it at the right times (number of times a day)
✔ Taking it with or without the right foods (empty stomach, with a meal, with or without dairy products)
✔ Taking it with or without other medications
✔ Taking it for the right amount of time (10 days vs. ongoing)

Each of these is observable, and together they will result in the goal of taking the medication properly.

Now look back at your specific goal. Did you include all the necessary behaviors? If so, it's time to move on to the next SMART skill. If not, make it more specific and then move on.

M onitor Your Progress

There are several ways to create a medication diary, or log, to monitor your progress. A wall calendar or The Chart will work just fine. Each day, simply write down the name of the medication, the time you took it, and the amount you took. Put the calendar or chart somewhere near the medication, such as in the bathroom.

The American Heart Association offers a free medication monitoring chart, which can be downloaded from the Internet at: http://www.americanheart.org/presenter .jhtml?identifier=92.

A rrange Your World for Success

There are so many opportunities to *not* take medication—from forgetting, to running out, to not having it with you at the proper time. These barriers all can be overcome by arranging your world for success. Here are some strategies that can help you arrange your environment to increase the chances of taking your medication at the right time and in the right amount.

✔ Take medication with daily activities, such as eating breakfast or brushing your teeth.

✔ Use a pillbox with separate compartments for each day. They are inexpensive and can be purchased at most pharmacies.

✔ Put reminders everywhere: on the fridge, in the bathroom, on your nightstand, at work. The more reminders the better.

✔ Plan ahead for travel by filling a separate pill box.

✔ Throw away medications that are not currently prescribed to you.

R ecruit a Support Team

Taking your medication safely and consistently will help keep you healthy. This has direct benefits to your spouse, partner, family, friends, co-workers, employer, community, and even your pets. Getting help from the people around you is well justified. One of the simplest actions you can take is to let everyone you are comfortable with or have a close relationship with know that you need to take your medication regularly. Ask them to remind you. They can check on you with e-mails or phone messages, or remind you in person.

 In addition to friends, family, and co-workers, you can create what we call a *medication support team*. Your team could include your doctor or nurse practitioner, a care manager if you are participating in a disease management program, and your pharmacist. Although they may not remind you to take your medication, they can play a critical role in helping you take it safely. Make sure all the members of your health care team know what medicines you are taking (both pre scription and over-the-counter), and always report side effects to them. Always check with your doctor before stopping or changing a medication.

Your pharmacy can also play a helpful role. Try to see the same pharmacist each time you fill or refill a prescription. You can ask her about taking over-the-counter med ications with your prescriptions, and she can help clarify possible interactions between medications and between certain kinds of food and medications.

With the help of your family, friends, co-workers, and medication support team, you will be able to make the changes in your habits and routines needed to stick with the medication regimen as it was prescribed.

ACTION TIP
The Basics of Managing a Chronic Illness

From diabetes to heart disease to asthma, chronic conditions affect over 40 million Americans. When you are trying to juggle medications, doctor's visits, and everything else that is involved in managing a chronic disease, changing your diet and exercising can easily become overwhelming. Despite this, some simple actions that will help you manage any chronic condition include:

✔ Learn everything you can about the illness. You don't have to do it all at once; gather the information you need over time.

✔ Stay healthy. Eating well, exercising regularly, and getting enough sleep will increase your ability to manage your condition.

✔ Stress can make your condition worse, so take time to relax each day.

✔ Ask your family, friends, and health care providers to help you.

✔ Follow your doctor's instructions, especially about how to take the medications for your illness.

T reat Yourself

Why should you treat yourself for taking your medication properly? Some medications will make you feel better, and when you feel better, you are being rewarded or "treated." This makes it easier to take the medication on a regular basis. An aspirin that makes a headache go away or an antacid that soothes your stomach have built-in rewards in that they relieve your symptoms.

However, the medications used to treat conditions such as high cholesterol and depression are not likely to make you feel better immediately. Because of this, taking them doesn't give you any noticeable reward. Some medications, such as certain antiviral agents for HIV-AIDS and chemotherapy for cancer, don't make you feel better immediately, and the side effects can make you feel worse. However, most people feel that taking these medications is valuable because they promote health in the long run. The challenge in taking medication for a long period of time is that it's easy to forget until it becomes a habit. This is where having a reward or treat schedule can be useful.

If you have to take medication daily for an indefinite period of time, you need to make sure you are rewarded for doing it. Much as with exercise or diet, simply pick a treat that you will give yourself after taking your medication as prescribed for a week, or even each day. Here are a few suggestions; the trick is to pick something that *you* feel is a treat.

✔ Treat yourself to a low-calorie dessert at the end of the week.
✔ Go out to a movie or rent a special movie.
✔ Put gold stars on your monitoring chart after each day of successfully taking your medication.
✔ Tell youself, "I'm doing a great job at taking my medicines."

While it seems simple enough, many people fail to develop good habits for taking medication. When you have turned the act of taking your medication into a habit, you won't have to worry about forgetting to take it and you will improve your health. In some cases, you might even save your life.

PART III

Get Help When You Need It

*E*ven with the best of intentions and the most carefully laid plans, we all get stuck from time to time when we're trying to change. While the circumstances and specific behaviors may differ from person to person, there seems to be a set of sticking points that most people run into. This section is designed to help you get past them.

You may not need this kind of help right now, and if you don't—good for you. However, if you find yourself struggling at any point to make the changes you need to or want to make, read the stories in this section. You'll see how we work with people struggling with the most common sticking points. This is how we help them break through the major blocks and move closer toward their goals.

11

When Life Gets Tough: Coaching Sessions with Drs. Klapow and Pruitt

You have everything you need to make changes in any health behavior. By now, you can say "information, motivation, and SMART skills" in your sleep. However, you may be thinking, "Easier said than done," and, in a way, you're right. Knowing what to change, wanting to change, and having the SMART skills will help you be successful in making behavioral changes, but you will probably face challenges along the way. Almost everyone does.

Sometimes it can be helpful to see how other people have overcome their problems. The stories below are from some of our clients who wanted to make changes in their daily health habits, but were having difficulty. Read about their struggles, their successes, and how our coaching tips helped them to get over some of these hurdles. Test yourself, too. Fill in the spaces provided with your own advice about how to make successful behavioral changes.

Marie: "I'm completely motivated to lose weight and get healthier, but this is not working. Why am I stuck?"

Marie is a married, 27-year-old woman who has recently undergone two major life events: She graduated with a degree in veterinary medicine and had her first child. While pregnant, Marie felt free from following any serious constraints about eating, and she enjoyed many foods she had previously banished from her diet. The combination of pregnancy and her unchecked food choices resulted in a gain of about 55 pounds during her pregnancy.

Marie closely watched the scale following the birth of her baby, expecting to lose the weight "naturally" from breastfeeding and resuming a more health-conscious diet. During the first 2 weeks she was thrilled to see that she was losing weight, but she became disappointed as time passed, because she couldn't lose more than 20 of the 55 pounds she had gained.

Marie knew she needed to eat a healthy diet, and she was aware of the importance of regular exercise. However, exercise had been a problem for Marie even before her pregnancy. She recalled going through phases during which she would exercise consistently for a few months, stop for a while, and then start again when her clothes became too tight. Marie wanted to incorporate exercise into her life permanently so she could feel good about her weight and be as healthy as possible. Having a baby made Marie take a lot of things more seriously. She was motivated to make some changes for her own health, and she also wanted to be healthy for her new child.

Marie read this book, completed the interactive exercises, and was ready to get started. She set a short-term goal of walking on her treadmill 3 days a week (Monday,

Wednesday, and Friday) for 30 minutes from 6:30 to 7:00
A.M. She met this goal the first week, but only walked 1 day
each during the second and third weeks. By the fourth
week she had completely stopped. We met with Marie to
find out what had gone wrong. Here's what she said:

> "I was eager to get going on my exercise program. I
> was really motivated to lose weight and dedicate
> myself to getting and staying healthy. I read your
> book and followed your advice. I set a goal that was
> clear and not too difficult. I cleared the stack of boxes
> from my treadmill and arranged my environment
> just as you suggested. I even had my daily reward
> built in—I was going to treat myself by taking the
> time to watch my favorite television talk show if I
> had walked on the treadmill earlier that morning. I
> did everything just as you said. The first week went
> just great. Then the second week, my son was up for
> 2 nights in a row, and I was simply too tired to do any
> exercise. By the third week, each morning just
> seemed to slip by, and although I did walk on one
> day, the rest of the week was crazy. By the fourth
> week, it seemed as if I thought about using the tread-
> mill every day, but for whatever reason, I just didn't
> do it. This is so frustrating. I really want to lose
> weight. I couldn't be more motivated. Why is it so
> easy to forget or to do just about anything else other
> than walk on that darned treadmill?"

We asked Marie to think about the three key questions:
Do you know what to do? Do you want to do it? Do you

know how to change your habits and routines? She knew she had to walk on the treadmill to get in shape; she clearly wanted to do it, but somehow it just wasn't happening. Marie said, "Yes, I know what to do; yes, I want to do it; and yes, I now know how to change my routine. Why am I still having a problem?"

Marie's use of the SMART skills seemed worthy of a closer look. Marie had set a specific and achievable goal, arranged her environment for success, and had decided on an easy way to treat herself for meeting her daily walking goal. That left two SMART skills that Marie didn't mention: monitoring progress and recruiting a support team.

We asked Marie about her support team. She was clear about her husband's support. "My husband is 100 percent behind me on this. He agreed to watch our son and has been encouraging." It sounded like Marie had a reasonably good support team in her husband, but what about monitoring? She said that she copied The Chart out of the book, but she admitted she didn't use it because it didn't seem necessary just to track 30 minutes of walking in her own home.

 If you were coaching Marie about what to do to increase her chances of being successful with using her treadmill, what tips would you give her?

_____

_____

Did you suggest that Marie monitor her progress? This SMART skill seems to be the one she had overlooked. The tendency to discount the power of monitoring is something we see all the time. Keeping a close watch on behavior is especially important for counting calories, reducing the number of cigarettes you smoke, or keeping track of a complicated workout routine. But when the behavior is something as simple as walking once a day, keeping track of it on paper seems a bit silly because it's so easy to remember if you did it or not.

However, this is where many people go wrong. Keeping track of your actions isn't only about remembering what you did. In fact, the power in monitoring what you do is that it increases the likelihood of your repeating the behavior. Marie had a specific and measurable goal. She had arranged her world and had support and a reward schedule, but she had no cue or reminder to walk on her treadmill each morning. There was nothing to demonstrate the progress she was making in meeting her goal.

Marie needed to think about changing her routine as a game of probabilities. She should be doing everything possible to increase her chances of *doing the behavior* (in this situation, walking on the treadmill) and decrease the chances that she won't. What happened to Marie is a great demonstration of the need for a *set* of skills—not just one or two—in order to maximize the chances of being successful in making lasting behavioral changes. The SMART skills seem so simple and straightforward that people often underestimate the impact each one can have on behavior.

Marie found it difficult to believe that *not* monitoring her progress was the reason she was struggling with her walking program. She needed to be reminded of the power of this SMART skill. Her monitoring chart should be placed in a highly visible location. When she sees it, Marie will be forced to make a conscious decision between walking on the treadmill or not. Without a reminder or cue in your environment, it's easy for old habits, routines, and thoughts to take over. If Marie has a monitoring chart on the refrigerator and notices it every time she passes by, she will be much more likely to get on the treadmill. After Marie tracks her progress for a week or two, and recognizes how much she's accomplished, it will be difficult to stop moving toward her goal.

Marie is one of the most motivated people we've met. She really wanted to lose weight and improve her health. Her story is a great example of the need for more than willpower, desire, or motivation to change behavior. It's easy to be motivated for a week or so, but motivation alone won't pull you through. It simply isn't enough to keep new behaviors going. *All* the SMART skills have to be included in your plan to ensure the best chance of success. Good health doesn't happen just because you really want it, but there isn't any magic involved, either.

Susan is experiencing "the Drift."

"I've tried this before and it doesn't work," she said. "There has to be a better way."

It seems to happen every year. On New Year's Eve, Susan sets the goal of getting in shape for the annual beach vacation she takes with her husband each summer. She knows the SMART skills and follows them closely, but by March, Susan is slipping back into her old patterns.

Susan is 56 years old. She is generally healthy, but over the past 10 years she has become less active and has gained about 20 pounds. She knows she needs to watch her diet more closely and exercise regularly, and every January she starts the year off with a bang. In fact, for the past 5 years, Susan has lost about 10 pounds every year between January and April by following a strict eating and exercise plan. She strives for perfection, and rarely has a day in which she doesn't meet her eating and activity goals. Susan says her problem is that no matter how motivated she seems to be in January, her motivation fades by March, and she just can't seem to hold on to the lifestyle changes into the summer months. Here's what Susan said when we met with her:

> "I'm at my wit's end. This happens every year. I start the year really motivated and make good progress, but everything seems to fade away by spring. I don't understand how I can lose weight by exercising and eating right, and then by spring, bingo, I'm back to square one and the weight

returns. I've tried this behavioral stuff so many times before. It just doesn't work."

Susan is experiencing a pattern that happens to a lot of people. They start out strong, apply all of the SMART skills, and have good success for a short period of time. Then, something happens and they begin to lose their motivation. A number of our clients tell us they feel just as Susan does—that they're back to "square one." Susan needed to hear the good news: Her problem can be identified and resolved.

 Although it may seem like "bingo" and back to "square one" to Susan, let's examine this a bit more closely. Susan agreed that it took several weeks to lose those 10 pounds and get in the routine of regular exercise. Also, she agreed that it was physically impossible to gain the 10 pounds she had lost in a day. Even if Susan were to stop the eating and exercising changes she was making, it would be at least a few weeks until she gained back all of the weight she had lost. Thus, she may have some time to heed a warning.

 If you were Susan's behavioral change coach, what would you suggest to help her sustain the gains she had made over the first 3 months? What seems to be happening to her?

Maybe Susan's problem isn't that the SMART skills "just don't work." Maybe she needs to review Chapter 5, where we discussed behavioral drift. Recall that "drift" describes slipping back into old, more familiar patterns of behavior. In Susan's case, after about 3 months of making behavioral changes, she was slipping back into her old ways of eating too much and exercising too little.

Susan considered the possibility that she might be experiencing behavioral drift. She also entertained the idea that the SMART skills might be effective if she kept doing them. Although Susan somewhat agreed with what we were saying, she clearly wasn't convinced. We forged ahead.

The good news for Susan was that her problem was easy to solve. She simply needed to catch herself drifting back into her old patterns. If she could use the "three-day rule" (see Chapter 5) to catch herself, she would be able to get back on track and meet her goal.

Susan wanted to know what was so important about 3 days. We told her this was her "red flag," a signal to stop and find out why she was getting off-track and not meeting her eating and activity goals. We emphasized that the beauty of the three-day rule was that it would allow her to end the backward slide and prevent any significant weight gain (remembering that no one can gain 10 pounds in 3 days). If Susan catches herself in the first three days of getting off-track and corrects her course, she will not regain the weight she's lost.

Although she understood the importance of the three-day rule, Susan still was concerned that her enthusiasm for sticking with her new behaviors seemed to fade fairly quickly, and that all seemed to be lost once it faded. For Susan, the solution was to catch problems early by being alert to the onset of behavioral drift *and* sustaining some level of motivation across time.

 What coaching tips would you give Susan about motivation and how to keep it going over time?

_____

_____

_____

_____

For most people, motivation for making behavioral changes tends to wax and wane. Motivation is dynamic over time, and as a result, it requires some ongoing attention. There are several effective strategies that will keep motivation going. One is to remind yourself frequently about your reasons for wanting to eat better or exercise more. Susan should take a minute to consider the following questions: How do you want to feel 5 years from today? How healthy do you want to be? How do you want to look? How physically fit do you want to be? She might benefit from writing her answers to these questions on a sheet of paper, so she can review them often to remind herself of the benefits of making healthy changes.

More motivational questions include: What are you doing today to become the person you had in mind when you started making lifestyle changes? What steps are you taking *right now* to ensure that you become that person? When we asked Susan, she said, "Those questions definitely make me think."

Susan can also think of motivation as self-perpetuating. By using the SMART skills, she can start a behavioral change cycle in which she initially has a level of motivation to make the desired changes. As she recognizes progress in an area (such as weight loss) her motivation will continue and increase because she likes the experience of success. As Susan continues to use the SMART skills, she will be able to maintain her motivation, and the positive cycle will perpetuate itself.

Doing these simple motivational exercises will remind Susan of why she started to make behavioral changes in the first place, and they will give her that little boost of motivation she needs to keep going. Motivation can build on itself, too. If Susan will catch problems early, stick with the SMART skills, and think about boosting her motivation along the way, she will prevent the drift from pulling her back into her old behavior patterns of eating to much and exercising too little.

Susan's frustration, expressed as "I've tried this before—behavioral stuff just doesn't work," is something we hear a lot. It's not that the SMART skills don't work—but that they work *only when you use them*. Instead, people initially have the motivation to change and they use the SMART skills. At some point, however, motivation declines and nothing is done to replenish it. Then, the SMART skills drop out and, eventually, old behavioral patterns re-emerge. This experience has a name: "behavioral drift" and drift is something we (and you) know how to address.

 All of us are at risk of reverting to old habits when we start making changes in our routines. Initially, we think: "That won't happen to me. I have the motivation to stick with it." In fact, behavioral drift is powerful, and if you think about it for a minute, it makes sense. If you've had a habit for 1, 5, or even 10 years, and then try to change it, wouldn't you expect to be pulled back into your long-standing, familiar patterns? The good thing about the concept of drift is that we slip back to our old ways, not suddenly. If we stay alert, we can catch drift early, reevaluate our motivational levels, and get back on track using the behavioral skills we have learned. The risk of drift will always be there, but the longer you stick with your new behaviors by using the SMART skills, the more motivated you will be and the less impact the drift will have.

Bill: "These basic principles and the SMART skills just don't apply to me. My problems are far more complicated."

Bill is a 45-year-old successful businessman, with a solid marriage and two small children. Throughout his early adult life, Bill was a dedicated athlete. He ran every day, lifted weights, ate a healthy diet, and focused a lot of attention on staying fit. Bill played football in college, but a serious knee injury during his senior year ended his athletic career.

Following his knee injury, Bill's lifestyle and conscientious health habits gradually changed. Following his marriage, he tried to stay fit by going to the gym. This seemed to work for a few years, but Bill began to slack off doing his regular exercise routine when he started working as a banker. At the same time, his healthy diet began to deteriorate. Slowly, over the course of 15 years, Bill went from being a physically fit, college athlete to a 45-year-old, obese man.

Bill went to his doctor for a physical and found out he has high cholesterol, borderline hypertension, and is in the beginning stage of Type 2 diabetes. He has developed mild degenerative arthritis in his knee—the one with the old injury. Bill told us:

"I'm falling apart. I'm 45 years old, in terrible shape, and I'm going downhill fast. I have to change everything. I need to eat differently, exercise regularly, start taking medication, and reduce the stress in my life. How the heck am I going to do all this? It's just too much to handle if I expect to keep working and take care of my family. I understand the principles, and I know the SMART skills, but my problems are more complicated. I need to make a lot of behavior changes—changes that involve every aspect of my life. I need more help than your basic principles and those simple behavior skills. My problems are too complicated."

Obviously, Bill had reached his limit both physically and emotionally. His body was telling him he could no longer keep up the same pace without some help. We talked about his need to change his health habits in the same way that you need to care for your car. Bill had been running his car at full speed for about 15 years without changing the oil, maintaining the brakes, keeping the transmission levels full, or lubricating the chassis. Now things were starting to fall apart.

Bill could relate to the car analogy. He went along with it, telling us he felt as if he was headed to the junkyard. He further stated that he knew how to fix his "car," but he didn't have the time or the skills to "overhaul" it. Because of this, he wakes up each day hoping the "car" will start. We let Bill know that many people find themselves in the same situation. Feeling overwhelmed is a common reaction to needing more than one lifestyle change. Bill was on a psychological merry-go-round. He knew he needed to make some significant changes in his life, but he didn't know where to start. As a result, his thoughts of needing to change just went around and around in his head, but he *never did anything about it.* We asked Bill if he felt "stuck," and he replied, "One hundred percent stuck." Bill was immobilized with thoughts and feelings about the changes he needed to make. He had no way to put his "transmission" into drive.

Despite being clear about the need to make several changes in his lifestyle, Bill needed to be challenged about his level of motivation. Was it possible that making the changes would be more trouble than it was worth? Bill admitted that sometimes he felt changing his health behavior was too much trouble, relative to the benefits to be gained, but he also knew he wanted to be healthy for his wife and children. He wanted to feel better, and he could see how his health problems were affecting his job and relationships. Bill told us he was scared. He was afraid he would fail if he tried to change.

We asked Bill to think about something other than his health. We wanted him to talk about things he understood, such as business and sports. Every business venture needs a strategy, and every competitive sport needs a game plan. Bill agreed that a person who has never run a business probably shouldn't start a multibillion dollar company, and a person who has never played a sport can't compete at the professional level. This was the case for Bill in dealing with his health. Other than his desire to change his behavior, he had no real plan; yet, he wanted to attempt a level of change he probably couldn't handle.

 If you were asked to help Bill tackle the behavior changes he wanted to make, what suggestions would you offer? How could he begin to make these changes?

Of course, Bill was capable of making all of the necessary behavior changes, but he was overwhelmed by thinking about them all at once. We emphasized the importance
of taking things one step at a time. Bill needed to re-think
his situation. He needed to make multiple changes: in his
diet, exercise program, medications, and stress management, and he needed to stick with them for the rest of his
life. These were Bill's ultimate goals, but we asked him to
focus on *one* thing he could do immediately that would
move him along the path to better health.

Bill told us he could start a diet or exercise program, but
that it seemed to be a huge and overwhelming task. He
believed it would never work. Because each of the changes
he needed to make seemed so big, Bill needed to scale back
even more. He needed to start with small, daily healthy
habits. We asked him to forget his exercise program for a
minute and focus instead on what other behaviors he could
do *this week* that would help him move toward his goals.

It was as if a light bulb had been turned on in his head.
"I could start doing the rehabilitation exercises for my
knee," he said. "Maybe I could talk with my wife about
what I should be eating to lose some of this weight. I know
I need to take my medications. Let's see. What else?"

Bill was on a roll but, once again, he was trying to take
on more changes than he could reasonably handle. If he

did his knee exercises this week and added some simple changes in his eating habits next week, by the third week he could consider the addition of some aerobic exercises to his routine. Bill had to have a clear goal and one that he was sure he could achieve. This would allow him to be on his way to success.

 However, Bill was stuck in a psychological "rut," and understandably feeling over whelmed because of the need to make multiple lifestyle changes. He knew what he needed to do, and he wanted to make the needed changes, but he just couldn't get started. This happened because he was focusing on the ultimate goals he was trying to achieve (weight loss, regular exercise, reduced stress, and medication compliance) without breaking them down into manageable behaviors. Bill could start small by doing his knee exercises, making some changes in his eating habits, and beginning a structured medication regimen.

Bill didn't need to accomplish everything immediately. He didn't need to do it *all*; he just had to start doing *something*. Achievable goals and small initial behavioral changes were all Bill needed to get the ball rolling.

Mike: "This is just common sense. What's the big deal about SMART skills?"

Mike is 57 years old. He's married, has two children, and works as an account executive for an advertising company. His son is beginning his junior year of college and his daughter just finished her freshman year. Now that his children are out of the house, he's decided it's time to get back in shape.

Mike has been relatively active throughout his life, but he's let his exercise habits slip and hasn't exercised consistently in about 10 years. An appendectomy, some prostate problems, and a busy lifestyle have left him about 15 pounds overweight. For the past few months, he hasn't been getting any physical activity that could be considered as exercise.

Mike's wife gave him this book because she's watched him struggle with trying to make lasting health behavior changes. She thinks his ideas about getting healthy are great, and he definitely talks a good line. She believes he is motivated to make some serious changes in his exercise and eating behavior. The problem is that Mike thinks this is all he needs: a little motivation and some common sense. In fact, after he read the book, he said, "What's the big deal? This is all common sense. I just need to get started."

Determined to get in shape, Mike joined the local gym and started watching what he eats. For 3 weeks he worked out every day and followed a strict diet. He lost 5 pounds, but he is exhausted and frustrated. He's hungry all the time, his knees hurt, and he's about to call it quits. Mike said:

> "This is ridiculous. I am working out like a madman, and I've only lost 5 pounds. I know these lifestyle changes are good for me, but I'm starting to feel like it's not worth it. It shouldn't be this difficult. I'm just about ready to give up. This is my pattern, isn't it?"

How would you respond to Mike if you were coaching him? Can you identify any problems with what he is doing?

_____

_____

_____

_____

_____

You probably recognized that Mike needs to revisit his goal in order to make sure it's clear, specific, and achievable. Helping him set a goal is a great place to start. Mike responded to our question about goals by indicating that he wants to lose 15 pounds and keep it off forever. He also wants to be in better overall physical shape.

Mike told us he anticipated it would take approximately a month to lose 15 pounds, but that he was hoping to lose the extra weight in less than 4 weeks by pushing himself to the limit. He thought he could be in good physical shape by then, too.

Mike's plan seemed in need of a reality check. It had taken quite a bit of time for him to get "out of shape"— about 10 years. How realistic was it to think he could get back into shape in less than 1 month? Was this an achievable goal? Was it clear and specific? As much as he wanted this experience to be over quickly, Mike had set the bar too high. He wasn't focused on observable behavior that could help him reach his goals to get more physical activity and change his eating habits in a specific manner. Because Mike didn't set a behavior goal that was specific—one that he was sure he could achieve—his chances of success were slim from the beginning.

Mike was adamant about his motivation and persistence. "I'm giving it everything I have. I want this to happen, and I know that I'll get there if I just push myself."

This is where many people (especially men) get it wrong. It's great to want to lose 15 pounds and get back in shape, but pushing too hard won't make the process go faster; instead, it will likely make you want to quit. Moreover, it's essential that Mike establishes realistic and reachable goals. If he doesn't, no matter how much motivation he has, he will run the risk of driving himself physically and mentally into the ground.

Mike honestly thought that losing 15 pounds was a good goal. At this point in our conversation, he appeared confused and asked us whether his goal might be unreasonable. Losing 15 pounds was not our concern, but Mike's unrealistic time frame and the fact that he wasn't tracking an observable behavior, such as jogging on the treadmill, could set him up for disappointment. Goals that can't be reached result in feelings of failure, and feelings of failure will reduce the chances of success in making positive lifestyle changes. Mike needed to break his goals into smaller, daily ones that were observable, measurable, and achievable.

We asked Mike to consider several questions about his behavioral targets, hoping that his answers would help him understand the importance of setting clear, specific, and achievable goals. How many days of the week was he going to exercise? For how long was he going to exercise? What specific activity was he planning to do? Where would he do the activity? What was he going to eat at each meal and where was he going to eat it? How many calories was he going to have daily? Was he going to follow a diet plan for every meal?

Mike immediately recognized that being specific would force him to look closely at what he was doing. By making his goals detailed, he could see them become measurable and more realistic. Finally, by having small daily and weekly goals instead of one big one, he could make the larger task much more manageable. In this way, short-term behavior goals can help Mike meet his long-term goals.

After his coaching sessions, Mike understood it was no surprise that he was tired, hungry, and frustrated. He decided that if he could focus on getting to the gym 4–5 days a week instead of 7, his behavior change strategy would be much more achievable. Mike finally had uttered the magic word, "achievable." This kind of "common sense" will get Mike where he wants to go.

 What other advice would you give Mike to help him be successful with changes in his exercise and eating habits?

_____

_____

_____

Hopefully, you advised him to add the remaining SMART skills into his plan. Monitoring, arranging his environment to help him be successful, recruiting support, and treating himself for meeting his goals will greatly increase his chances of getting into shape and losing 15 pounds. In fact, he *will* be successful if he follows all of these guidelines.

Finally, Mike is right that the SMART skills are common sense. It's not as if people haven't heard them before. Behavioral skills to help people change have been around for years, and they *are* simple and straightforward. However, thinking of the SMART skills only as "common sense" diminishes their power and discounts their potency. Mike is a great example of dismissing something that "everyone knows" and struggling with behavior changes as a result. Putting common sense into action is the key, and it starts with knowing how to set a realistic goal.

Donna: "I understand the formula and the SMART skills. I want to be healthy. I just need some motivation to exercise."

Donna is 40 years old and just beginning to feel the physical effects of getting older. She works full-time as a medical assistant for a busy primary care practice. She is a single mother of a 12-year-old son, and says that he is her top priority. Between his needs, her career, and a long commute to the office, Donna hasn't been able to fit exercise into her daily routine. She *knows* exercise is important to her overall health; she *wants* to be healthy, and she understands that exercise will help her feel better and keep her weight in check. Donna says her problem is a lack of motivation.

 If you were coaching Donna and advising her as to what to do about her problem, what would you say? What would you recommend as the next step?

_____

_____

_____

_____

_____

You may have noted that Donna does have *some* motivation. She stated that she wants to be healthy, and she recognizes the benefits of exercising. How could she take advantage of this? Does she need to examine the costs and benefits of exercise? Perhaps you advised Donna to get started on some type of activity program, even if it was a small beginning. If you suggested that the motivation she currently expressed is enough to get started—great! If Donna can leverage even a small amount of motivation to begin a behavior change program, she may discover that her motivation to continue will increase as she progresses toward her goal.

Donna didn't buy into the strategy of using what she already has to get started. She still didn't understand how she could find the time to exercise, given her commitments and responsibilities. How could she possibly fit one more thing into her schedule? She described feeling defeated before even starting an exercise plan: "Where will I find the motivation to do this—I have to get more motivated." Donna spoke as if motivation was something she could buy off the shelf or find on the Internet. She thought if she just had enough motivation, she would succeed. Now, if she could only locate it.

We thought maybe we could help Donna *locate* some motivation. Upon questioning her a bit more about her motivation with regard to exercise and the benefits she might experience, she described several more advantages: "I can lose weight, feel better, look better, be healthier, fit into my clothes, feel better about myself, and feel like I have some control over my life." This was a long list of benefits. Her list of drawbacks was shorter: "It will take time and energy." On balance, she agreed that exercising had a lot more benefits than not exercising.

When asked to put a number to her level of motivation, Donna rated her motivation to exercise at four on a ten-point scale. This number was relatively low, but clearly she has *some* level of motivation to change her exercise habits. She was surprised when we told her that this level of motivation was adequate to get started.

 How would you suggest Donna move forward, given that her motivation is enough to initiate a change in her behavior?

_____

_____

_____

_____

_____

If you recommended that Donna begin with setting a clear goal for exercise, one she is certain she can achieve, you have provided great advice. Did you suggest that she start small? Because Donna is not exercising at all, anything she does will be a big improvement. The point is to use the little bit of motivation that she has to start doing *something*. Starting small will increase her chances of success, and the experience of success will increase her motivation. Remember, motivation is self-perpetuating, and a small amount is all Donna needs to get started. Of course, Donna also needs to use the remainder of the SMART skills to ensure long-term success. She knows all of the SMART skills and can recite them without difficulty.

What would you suggest to Donna if she needed any help with the SMART skills? What does she need to do to monitor her progress? How would you recommend that Donna arrange her world for success, recruit a support team, and treat herself?

_____

_____

_____

_____

_____

 Achieving success is simply a matter of putting the SMART skills into play. Donna had enough motivation to get going with a behavior change plan. She didn't have to do a lot of exercise; she just needed to do some. Even a small amount of activity—such as walking for 30 minutes, 2 days a week—was a big improvement, and Donna finally began to experience the benefits she expected from getting more physical activity.

12
Action Tips for Special Situations

Get a Grip on Stress

We all experience stress at one time or another. What can you do when the pressures of life become too much? Stress has a way of building up to the point that you feel overwhelmed. The trick to managing it is to have a game plan. Try these suggestions:

✔ Make a list of the stressful situations in your life. Put a checkmark next to the ones you can change. Cross out the ones you can't. This will help you focus on what you can do versus what you can't.

✔ Don't let stressful thoughts grow bigger than the situation warrants. Take a look at the situations on your list. Can you think differently about some of them so they feel less stressful?

✔ Pay attention to your stress levels during the day. Every hour or so, take a minute to breathe deeply and collect your thoughts.

✔ Eat healthy, exercise regularly, and get enough rest. As hard as this seems, it will make you feel better.

Plan ahead and take control when life gets crazy.

Help Your Children Lead More Active Lifestyles

With cable television, video games, and the Internet, it's no wonder many children don't get enough exercise. Here is how you can help them become more physically active.

✔ Ask them to list specific activities they can do for a set amount of time. Maybe it's kicking a soccer ball for 15 minutes, shooting baskets, or playing on a swing set.
✔ Use a calendar to help them keep track of how much exercise they get each day.
✔ Establish new routines, such as having them exercise before they watch television. They may resist at first, but they'll come around because exercising will make them feel good.
✔ Just as you reward your kids for good grades, reward them for sticking with their new health habits.

You need to set a good example. If *you* don't exercise, it sends a negative message to your children. These tips will help you establish more active routines for your children. And who knows—you may become more active as well.

Beating Road Rage

We've all heard about road rage and the deadly consequences of letting our emotions spin out of control. With
our busy schedules and more of us on the road, it's easy for
a little frustration to turn into full-blown road rage. Keeping your emotions in check is the key. Try these helpful
tips:

✔ Focus on your breathing while driving, and make sure
  it's slow and steady. The more regulated your breathing, the more relaxed you'll feel.
✔ Loosen your grip on the steering wheel and drop your
  shoulders to help reduce muscle tension.
✔ Use music to regulate your mood. Listening to slow-
  paced relaxing music will reduce tension without your
  even trying.
✔ Set realistic time expectations—if you're in a hurry and
  late, you are almost guaranteed to be tense. Allow
  enough time to get where you're going.

Driving can be a frustrating experience, but it doesn't
need to be a deadly one. Stay in control of your emotions
and you'll be safer on the road.

Heart-Healthy Actions

Cardiovascular disease is the nation's number one killer. If
you want to reduce your chances of heart disease here's
what to do:

✔ Maintain a healthy weight using the concepts in this book to help your motivation level.

✔ Manage your blood pressure and cholesterol. Get them checked often. Sometimes your local pharmacy will do this for free or at a low cost.

✔ Reduce salt intake; don't use it in cooking or add it at the table.

✔ Exercise.

✔ Don't smoke. Quit immediately if you do!

✔ Lower your stress levels, when necessary. Take 10–15 minutes to relax your mind and body by using, for example, deep breathing or yoga exercises, listening to soothing music, taking a hot bath or shower, or rearranging your environment—take a walk if a situation becomes overly stressful.

Will doing these things today prevent heart disease? No, not in one day, but it is a start, and sometimes that's all you need.

Getting over Gym Phobia

Let's face it, going to a gym or health club can be a little intimidating, so here are some tips to help you ease into the gym experience.

✔ First, find a gym or club that is close to home or work. The closer it is, the more likely you are to go.

✔ Take a tour and ask as many questions as you want before you join. Make sure it's the right gym for you.

✔ Take advantage of free personal training or use a trainer for a short time. This is a great way to become familiar with the equipment and develop a work routine.

✔ Finally, if you're feeling a little self-conscious, train at "off–peak hours" when the gym is less crowded.

Remember every person in the gym was unsure of herself the first time she walked through the door. The longer you stick with it, the more comfortable you will become.

Dealing with Holiday Stress

The holidays are supposed to be a time of joy and bliss, but for many people the preparations and obligations lead to added stress. Here are some tips to help you keep your holiday stress in check:

✔ Be realistic about the holidays. They don't need to be perfect to be joyous. Remind yourself that there will be good times and bad times.

✔ Remember that it's okay to feel stressed, sad, and angry during the holidays. Feeling bad doesn't mean the holidays are ruined.

✔ Slow down and prioritize your activities. You can't attend every party, buy every gift, cook every meal, and visit every relative. Write down everything you plan to do during the holidays, and then read the list out loud. Is it a reasonable list? If not, start crossing things off.

✔ Pay attention to your health. Get plenty of sleep, try to eat right, and exercise when you can. Your holiday won't be joyous if you are sick or overstressed.

We all want the holidays to be a happy time. By having realistic expectations and not overextending, you will keep your stress levels in check and increase your enjoyment.

Managing the Holiday Blues

The holidays are a time of joy for most people. However, holiday time can also mean a bout of the "blues." Here are some tips that should help:

✔ Set realistic expectations for the holidays. As special as they are, they will not erase all of your past problems.
✔ Remember that it's okay not to feel festive all of the time. If you are feeling down, just let others know.
✔ Take some time for yourself. Plan activities that you enjoy, and spend time with family or close friends.
✔ Be sure to get plenty of sleep, eat healthy meals, stay active, and limit your intake of alcohol.

What if someone you love has the blues?

✔ Try to involve that person in holiday activities, but don't be forceful.
✔ Be a good listener. Remember that the holidays can be a tough time for some people, and letting them talk about it may be all they need.

The *good* news is that, for most people, holiday blues are temporary. However for some people, the holidays can bring on the more serious condition of clinical depression. If you or someone you know doesn't shake the blues after a few weeks, its time to talk with your doctor or a mental health professional.

Holiday Spending

For many people holiday shopping results in heavy debt. Shopping is a behavior that often spins out of control. Here are some tips that will help you better manage your spending:

- ✔ Make a list of the people you are going to shop for and write down the total amount that you are going to spend on each of them.
- ✔ Take cash when you go shopping and leave the credit cards at home. Also, make sure you give yourself enough time to shop so that you won't be pressured into making last-minute impulse purchases. While you are shopping, write down every purchase and the price next to each person's name on your list.
- ✔ Make yourself accountable by letting one other person know how much you have budgeted. Being accountable to someone else will help you maintain control.
- ✔ Set aside some funds as an incentive for staying within your budget. You can purchase something for yourself or give it to charity.

With a bit of planning you can reduce the stress of overspending and really enjoy the holiday shopping experience.

Talking about Emotional Problems

Everyone feels sad or anxious at one time or another. But what do you do when those feelings start getting the best of you? You may feel awkward when talking with your doctor, but emotional problems are just as serious and treatable as physical problems. To make it easier, talk with your doctor about your emotional symptoms just as you would about physical symptoms. Tell your doctor when the symptoms started, how often they occur, and how the symptoms are impacting your daily life

Make sure you discuss and understand your treatment options. This might mean psychotherapy, medication, or a follow-up visit. This strategy will make the conversation easier, but the most important action you can take is to follow through with treatment. If left untreated, emotional symptoms can get much worse.

Being a Caregiver

Nearly 21 percent of Americans provide care for a chronically ill or disabled loved one over the age of 18. But caregiving can take a toll on the mind and body. Taking care of your own health is one of the most important things you can do. If you become ill, who will do the caregiving? Here are some simple ways to make sure you care for yourself:

✔ Stay healthy. Make sure you eat well, get enough sleep, and exercise each day.
✔ Keep a journal of your thoughts and feelings. It's a great release for your emotions.
✔ Do one activity that you enjoy every day.
✔ Set aside time to be with others for an evening out or having friends over to visit.
✔ Ask for help from a friend, family member, or professional organization. You don't have to do this alone.

You may feel guilty about focusing on yourself, but these efforts will help you feel better and give you the strength you need to be the best caregiver possible.

13

You CAN Do This

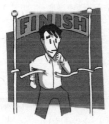

There you have it! As we promised at the beginning of this book, you now have everything you need to make *any* lifestyle change you desire. Stop for just a moment and think about this, because it's important. You now have a foundation for living a healthier life. You may choose not to use it from time to time, but whenever you want to change a health-related behavior you have the basic principles and skills you need.

Think about all of the health-related behaviors that you could improve using the ideas in this book. Having The What, The Want, and SMART skills to accomplish The How can empower you to change your life. More importantly, when you make changes in your lifestyle, you will be able to stick with it.

Life gets in the way of our intentions and plans, so having a strategy to stay the course is critical. You will stray from your healthy lifestyle from time to time, and sometimes you will feel your motivation slipping, but you can remind yourself that when it's time to get back on track you have everything you need. Living SMART is not about being perfect, it's about making the right choices and engaging in the right behaviors more days than not. Remember the three-day rule. If you skip a workout or cheat on your diet, you have made one "bad" choice and engaged in one "bad" behavior, but tomorrow you can use the SMART skills to get moving again in a positive direction. We're confident you will do a great job. Congratulations, you are on your way to living a healthier life.

Joshua C. Klapow, Ph.D.
Sheri D. Pruitt, Ph.D.

A
Charts for Change

This section includes useful information and copies of some of the charts in the book, as well as additional interactive exercises to help you reach your goals. These can easily be photocopied. For additional resources, including many you can download, visit the Living SMART web page at www.livingsmart.diamedicapub.com.

The Chart: The What, The Want, and The How

My health behavior is: _____ (be specific)

I will practice my behavior _____ days per week.

My short-term goal is _____.

My long-term goal is _____.

I will give myself _____(treat)

on the following schedule:

_____ (how often).

In addition to giving myself _____, when I

complete _____ (number of days, weeks, or months),

I will give myself a bonus treat of _____.

SUN	MON	TUE	WED	THU	FRI	SAT

Interactive Exercises to Increase Your Motivation

These fast and easy exercises will help you increase your motivation levels. They can be done any time you feel your motivation slipping. Doing them from time to time will help you stay motivated.

Forecasting Your Future

What if you aren't sure you are motivated enough to make a change? Stop for a moment and think about your future. If you don't change your health habits, will you still be here 5 years from now? Will you be able to work, go on vacation, and enjoy life? Will you be able to do the things you want to do? Your future and your ability to function in that future are determined in large part by what you do today, tomorrow, and the next day. Ask yourself these questions and write down the answers:

What health behavior are you most likely to change? ____
_____.

What made you select this particular behavior? _____
_____.

How would you feel if you were to make this change? ___
_____.

What else would be different about you? _____
_____.

What behavior have you been able to change in the past?
_____
_____.

Next, imagine yourself 5 years from now:

If my behavior stays the same, I will feel _____

_____.

If I keep doing exactly what I am doing now, I will look

_____

_____.

If I don't change a thing, my health will be _____

_____.

Imagine your loved ones 5 years from now:

If my behavior stays the same, it will affect my loved ones by _____

_____.

If my behavior stays the same, my loved ones may react by

_____

_____.

By taking the time to answer these questions, most of you will be reminded of why you set out to make changes in the first place. Simple as it seems, this little reminder can really boost your level of motivation. So, if you ever find your motivation slipping, repeat this exercise.

Weighing the Pros and Cons of Change

There are advantages and disadvantages to changing any behavior, and it's important to consider both when you're trying to get motivated. For example, think about eating ice cream every night. This is a behavior that you might want to change because you want to lose weight. Consider the pros and cons of continuing or stopping this behavior:

Behavior: Eating ice cream every night

Continuing the Behavior:	
Pros	**Cons**
If I continue eating ice cream, I will continue to enjoy the cool, creamy, sweet taste that I love so much.	If I continue eating ice cream every night, I'll keep gaining weight.
Changing the Behavior:	
Pros	**Cons**
If I cut down on ice cream, I'll feel more in control of my eating habits.	If I reduce my ice cream intake, I'll feel deprived.

Next, apply the same "pros and cons" strategy to determine the advantages and disadvantages of making this particular behavioral change.

Behavior I Want to Change: _____.

Continuing the Behavior:	
Pros	Cons

Changing the Behavior:	
Pros	Cons

Is Making This Change Important?

How important is making a specific behavior change? Use the scales below to rate how important it is for you to make the behavioral change you're considering and how confident you are that you will succeed:

1. How important is it that I make the change?

1	2	3	4	5	6	7	8	9	10

Not
important

Extremely
important

2. What would make this behavioral change more important?

_____

_____

3. Am I confident I can make the change?

1	2	3	4	5	6	7	8	9	10

Not confident
at all

Extremely
confident

4. What would make you more confident?
(Circle yes or no.)

More information?	Yes	No
Smaller changes?	Yes	No
Help making the change?	Yes	No
More reasons to change?	Yes	No

By answering these questions, you have probably discovered a number of reasons for changing or refusing to change an unhealthy behavior. You've probably realized that your emotions play a significant role in your decision to make the change. Thinking about changing a behavior can bring up a variety of emotions, including anger, fear of failure, and anxiety. While change can be difficult and stressful, consider the consequences of *not* changing. What are you doing today to become the healthy person you envision yourself being in the future? How long can you afford to wait before making the change?

Tips for Defeating Negative Thoughts

You can be sailing along and then—all of a sudden—it happens. You experience some small setback in your diet, exercise program, or management of your blood pressure, and then the flood of negative thoughts comes. This type of thinking will dampen your motivation, but it doesn't have to mean the end of your success. Here is a simple strategy for managing negative thoughts:

1. *Catch yourself when you experience a negative thought.*
   Negative thoughts most often occur following a slip-up. Take a minute to write down your answers to the following questions: What's going through my mind? What are my thoughts? Maybe they are something like: "I have no self-control" or "I'm not disciplined enough to do this."

2. *Turn the thought into an action.*

Once you've caught the negative thought and written it down, repeat it out loud, but imagine someone else is saying it to you. Imagine, for example, that someone said: "You have no self-control" or "You're just not disciplined enough." By picturing someone else saying the words, you will be more likely to stick up for yourself. This takes us to the third step.

3. *Defend yourself.*

Do you really lack self-control? Chances are this negative thought isn't 100 percent accurate. Think about the times when you have shown self-control, and write down as many examples as you can to prove that this negative thought is not true. Also, think about other explanations for why you slipped up this time.

This exercise won't keep you from having negative thoughts, and it won't prevent occasional slip-ups. It will, however, keep one slip-up and one negative thought from taking over and ruining your efforts. By catching your negative thoughts and defeating them, you will be able to keep your motivation levels up and stay on track.

SMART Skills

Using the SMART skills can make the difference between people who make health changes and stick with them, and people who try but don't succeed. Here are two examples:

Exercise:

The five things you need to do if you want to become more physically active are:

S *et a clear, achievable goal.*

Be sure your health goal is specific and that it can be measured. For example, "I will walk 30 minutes, 3 days a week" is a clear, specific, and measurable goal. Start small—choose a goal you can accomplish, and then build on your success.

M *onitor your progress.*

Track your progress using a simple calendar so that you have a visible "report card" of your health behavior changes over time. Put an "x" on each day that you meet your goal. If you're not accomplishing what you planned, you can check the calendar for patterns and adjust your behavior. Use The Chart in Chapter 6 to keep track of your progress; for example, to record the number of minutes (in 5-minute increments) that you exercise each day. Watch your progress and be proud of yourself!

A *rrange your world for success.*

Putting reminders to exercise in your car, office, refrigerator door, and bathroom mirror can help you succeed. Put your gym bag in your car so you have everything you need for a workout. Post a picture of a walker or a runner above your desk to remind you what you're working toward. Put your monitoring form in a place you will see every day, such as the refrigerator door or the bathroom mirror.

R ecruit a support team.

Enlist the help of others. Let the people who want to see you succeed know what you're trying to achieve. Consider your family, friends, and work colleagues as your potential support team. *Ask* them to support your efforts in meeting your activity goals, and to join you in celebrating your success. They will be happy to let you know you're doing a great job!

T reat yourself.

Reward yourself every time you do the health behavior you have targeted. Treat yourself after every walk, every gym session, or every time you meet your activity goals. Select a "treat" that is important to you, readily available, and not costly. A hot shower with special soap, 10 minutes of alone time, or a chat with your exercise partner are some good examples of treats. Treats are especially important when you are starting a new health behavior—you can phase them out over time as the new behavior becomes automatic.

Eating Behaviors:

If you want to change your eating habits, the same five skills look like this:

S et a clear, achievable goal.

Be sure your eating goal is specific and is something you can measure. For example, "I will eat five servings of fruits and vegetables a day" is an example of a clear, specific, and measurable goal. Start small—choose a goal you can accomplish, then build upon your success.

M onitor your progress.

Keep track of what you do. You can use a simple calendar to monitor your behavioral changes over time. Put an "x" on each day that you meet your goal. Look for patterns and make adjustments if you're not accomplishing what you planned. Use the Monitoring Form that you can download from our Web site to track your actions each day. Watch your progress and feel proud!

A rrange your world for success.

Create reminders for healthy eating all around you. Put your monitoring form in a place you see every day, such as the refrigerator door or your bathroom mirror. Make it easy to eat healthy foods by always having them available. A great way to do this is to take your lunch to work.

R ecruit a support team.

Enlist the help of others. Let those who want to see you succeed know what you're trying to achieve. Consider your family, friends, and work colleagues as your potential support team. *Ask* them to support your efforts in meeting your eating goals and to join you in celebrating your success. They will be happy to let you know you're doing a great job!

T reat yourself.

Reward yourself every time you do the eating behavior you have targeted. Select a "treat" that is important to you, readily available, and not costly. A low-calorie beverage, a few minutes of alone time, or simply telling yourself you're doing a great job are some good examples of treats. Rewarding yourself is especially important in the beginning, when you are starting a new health behavior—you can phase them out over time.

You can apply this same set of skills to any health behavior you want to change—or *any* behavior at all, for that matter.

Set a Goal

Setting an Exercise Goal

Did you know that even a small amount of exercise can improve your health and fitness? Regular exercise can reduce your risk of a number of health problems, including chronic pain, diabetes, and stress. Your overall well-being can improve significantly after making even small lifestyle changes.

People who are successful at starting new health habits begin with clear, achievable goals: specific, measurable, and observable. Here are some examples of good and not so good goals for exercising:

"Exercise More" is a nice idea, but not specific enough to be a good goal.

"Walk 5 miles a day" is specific and measurable, but probably not realistic if you aren't already walking regularly.

"Walk 30 minutes every day at lunchtime" is more attainable, but what if you have an extra busy day or the weather is sometimes bad at noon?

"Walk 30 minutes, 5 days a week" is specific, measurable, and observable, and it is something you can likely achieve.

Here are some questions to ask yourself in order to help you set a behavioral goal.

1. This week, what do you specifically want to achieve?
- Which activity do you want to do?
  Walking Running Biking Swimming
  Other_____
- How much time do you want to spend exercising on the days that you exercise?
  5 minutes 10 minutes 15 minutes 20 minutes
  Half Hour
- How many days a week do you want to exercise?
  3 days 4 days 5 days 6 days 7 days

2. Is your goal behavior something you can see and measure?
  A good goal can be measured and charted so that you will know if you met it.
- How will I keep track of my exercise this week?
  chart diary calendar palm pilot other

3. Is your goal for the week realistic?
  A good goal is something you are likely to achieve. Make sure you have the time and everything you need to achieve it. Many people have busy days, and you may need to plan carefully to fit exercise into your schedule.

My activity goal for this week is:

The activity: _____

The number of days per week: _____

The number of minutes per day: _____

Can I meet this goal? _____

Setting an Eating Goal

Whether you want to eat more fruits and vegetables, eat fewer calories, reduce your portion size, or cut out sweets, the goal you select is critical for your success.

People who are successful at starting new health habits begin with clear, achievable goals. Your goal should be specific, something that can be measured or counted, and something that can be seen if another person was watching you. Here are some examples of good and not so good goals for changing eating habits:

"I want to eat a healthier diet" is a nice idea, but not specific enough to be a good goal.

"I want to eat five servings of fruits and vegetables every day" is specific and measurable, but probably not realistic if you haven't been eating fruits and vegetables at all.

"I want to eat two servings of fruits and vegetables every day at lunchtime" is more attainable, but what if you have an extra busy day and cannot find healthy food?

"I want to eat two servings of fruits and vegetables, 3 days a week" is specific, measurable, and observable, and it is something you can likely achieve.

Here are some questions to ask yourself that will help you set a behavioral goal about eating.

1. This week, what do you specifically want to achieve?
  - Which eating habit do you want to change?
    more fruits/vegetables   fewer calories
    reduce fast food   limit sweets   other_____
  - How many days per week do you want to target for changing your eating habits?
    2 days   3 days   5 days   7 days   other_____

2. Is your eating goal something you can see and measure?
    A good goal behavior is something that can be measured or counted, and charted so you will be able to track your progress.
  - How will I keep track of my eating behavior this week?
    monitoring chart   food diary   calendar
    palm pilot   other_____

3. Is your goal realistic for this week?
    A good goal is something you are likely to achieve. Make sure that you have everything you need to meet the goal you've set with regard to eating behaviors. We all have busy days and unexpected interruptions. You may need to plan carefully to fit your new eating habits into your schedule.

My eating goal for this week is: _____
The specific eating habit I want to change is: _____

The number of days per week I will work on my eating habits: _____

Can I meet this goal? _____

Monitor Your Progress

Self-Monitoring Form for Exercise

Use a chart like the one below to keep track of your progress as you begin your new exercise routine. A calendar can serve the same purpose. Remember that monitoring is a very powerful SMART skill. This chart is marked for someone who has a goal of walking 10 minutes per day the first week, 15 minutes per day the second week, and 20 minutes per day the third week.

Minutes	M	T	W	Th	F	S	S	M	T	W	Th	F	S	S	M	T	W	Th	F	S	S
70																					
65																					
60																					
55																					
50																					
45																					
40																					
35																					
30																					
25																					
20																					
15																					
10																					
5																					

Determine your activity goal for the first few weeks. It's a good idea to identify this in some way on your monitoring form. Next, place a check mark in the boxes representing the number of minutes that you exercise each day. In the example above, if you started a walking program on Monday, and you walked 10 minutes, you could put a check mark in the 5-minute box and one in the 10-minute box. If you fulfill your goal, all of the colored boxes will have a check at the end of the week.

Use the second page of the download version available at **www.livingsmart.com** to continue to track your exercise over time. Make as many copies as you need, so you can keep track of the behavior over time.

Self-Monitoring Form for Eating

Week 1							Week 2							Week 3							Week 4						
M	T	W	T	F	S	S	M	T	W	T	F	S	S	M	T	W	T	F	S	S	M	T	W	T	F	S	S

Use a chart like this one to keep track of your progress as you begin your new eating habits. A calendar can serve the same purpose. Remember to record each time you do your target behavior. You can keep track of calories, or use a simple check mark for breakfast, lunch, or dinner that meets your eating goal. Monitoring is a very powerful SMART skill.

Determine your eating goal for the first few weeks. It's a good idea to identify this in some way on your monitoring form. Next, place a check mark in the boxes each day that you met your goal. For example, if you start a new eating habit on Monday, and you took a low-calorie, healthy lunch to work for five days, then you could check each box in the middle row for Monday, Tuesday, Wednesday, Thursday, and Friday.

You can make as many copies of this monitoring form as you need to keep track of the behavior over time, or you can create another form that works better for you—whatever best allows you to keep track of your eating behavior.

Arrange Your World for Success

Arranging your world for success is all about taking control of your life in small but powerful ways. Making and sticking with changes will become easier and easier if you can break down small barriers. List on the form below (or print it from our Web site) a health behavior that you want to change *other than exercise*, such as eating healthy food, quitting smoking, getting more sleep, or remembering to take your medication. Then, list the things you can do to set up the world around you to help you be successful. As we're sure you'll see, with a little thought you can be successful in arranging your world to help you meet your goals.

Behavior I want to change: _____

Ways I can arrange my environment to support this change:

1. _____

2. _____

3. _____

4. _____

5. _____

Treat Yourself Checklist

Behaviors that are rewarded are more likely to be repeated. This is a well-known fact of human behavior that you can use to your advantage. Give yourself a "treat" each time you perform an activity or behavior that you want to continue. Treats can be short-term and long-term. Short-term rewards might include 10 minutes of alone time, watching the sunset at the end of your walk, or telling yourself "great job." Long-term rewards can include new walking shoes or workout clothes. Treats need to be meaningful to you! Plan them in advance so that you know what you're working toward, and choose ones that will reward your target behavior.

Make a list of short-term rewards:

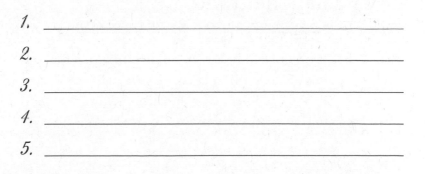

1. _____

2. _____

3. _____

4. _____

5. _____

Make a list of long-term rewards:

1. _____

2. _____

3. _____

4. _____

5. _____

I will give myself_____ as a reward for each time I do
_____ physical activity. (These treats will help
a behavior get started).

When I meet my activity goals for one month, I will treat
myself with _____.

In addition to giving myself _____ (reward), if I
complete _____ (number of days, weeks, or months) of
_____ (health behavior), I will give myself a
bonus treat of _____
(choose a bonus reward).

Getting Back on Track

What If... Exercise

This "What If..." list will help you target situations that are
likely to lead to behavioral drift. The details will be different
for each health-related behavior, but the process and general topics are the same. Here are some common examples.

✔ What if the weather is bad and I can't exercise outside?

✔ What if we go out to dinner and they don't have the foods on my diet?

✔ What if we are traveling and I can't get to bed at a reasonable hour?

✔ What if I go to a bar and someone offers me a cigarette?

✔ What if my schedule changes and I can't do my relaxation exercises in the morning before work?

✔ What if my motivation levels decrease?

✔ What if the rewards I am using no longer work?

✔ What if I am sick or injured, and unable to exercise, prepare certain meals, or take my scheduled medications?

✔ What if my change partner is no longer available?

✔ What if my supporters are no longer available?

List three or more "What If" scenarios that might affect your success in achieving your health goals.

1. _____

2. _____

3. _____

4. _____

5. _____

These situations will not necessarily cause behavioral drift, but they are good warning signs. Therefore, the longer the list is, the better. If you can anticipate it, you can plan for it—and if you can plan for it, you will know how to deal with it.

Three-Day Rule Pledge

Use this worksheet to help you stick with the three-day rule. Copy it from this book (or download it from our Web site), fill it out, and post it where you can see it regularly.

Three-Day Rule Pledge

If I stop the actions I have set out to reach my goals for a period of three days, for ANY reason, I pledge to sit down and do the following:

1. Write down why I have stopped.
2. Write down what I need to do to get started again.
3. Write down the exact date I plan to start again.
4. Post the start-up date on the refrigerator or some other location that I can easily see.

Date:

Signature:

B

Additional Resources

Nutrition:

U.S. Department of Agriculture:
www.health.gov/dietarybooklines
    Informative booklets, *Guidelines* and *Using the Dietary Guidelines*, are available from the Consumer Information Center. Order on-line or call (888) 878-3256.

American Dietetic Association: www.eatright.org
(800) 877-1600.

Exercise:

The President's Council on Physical Fitness and Sports:
www.fitness.gov or call (202) 690-9000.

American Heart Association: www.americanheart.org
(800) 242-8721.

Smoking:

American Lung Association: www.lungusa.org or call
(800) 548-8252.

The Foundation for a Smoke Free America
www.anti-smoking.org or call (310) 471-4270.

Substance Abuse:

National Institute on Drug Abuse: www.drugabuse.gov or call (800) 729-6686.

Cancer Prevention:

American Cancer Society: www.cancer.org or call (800) ACS-2345 (866-228-4327 for TTY). Cancer Information Specialists available 24 hours a day.

Centers for Disease Control: www.cdc.gov/cancer or call (888) 842-6355.

HIV/STD Prevention:

National Prevention Information Network: www.cdcnpin.org or call (800) 458-5231.

Diabetes:

National Diabetes Education Program: www.ndep.nih.gov
    Call (800) 438-5383 to order education materials for consumers and healthcare providers.

Heart Disease:

American Heart Association: www.americanheart.org or call (800) AHA-USA-1 or (800) 242-8721.

Obesity:

U.S. Department of Health and Human Services: www.smallstep.gov or call (877) 696-6775.

Index